Return from Madness

Psychotherapy with People Taking the New Antipsychotic Medications and Emerging from Severe, Lifelong, and Disabling Schizophrenia

KATHLEEN DEGEN, M.D.,
AND
ELLEN NASPER, Ph.D.

JASON ARONSON INC.
Northvale, New Jersey
London

Production Editor: Judith D. Cohen

This book was set in 11 pt. Bem by TechType of Ramsey, New Jersey and printed and bound by Book-mart Press of North Bergen, New Jersey.

Library of Congress Cataloging-in-Publication Data

Degen, Kathleen.
    Return from madness : psychotherapy with people taking the new antipsychotic medications and emerging from severe, lifelong, and disabling schizophrenia / by Kathleen Degen and Ellen Nasper.
        p.   cm.
    Includes bibliographical references and index.
    ISBN 1-56821-625-4 (alk. paper)
    1. Schizophrenia— Treatment.   2. Clozapine.   3. Group psychotherapy.   I. Nasper, Ellen Deborah.   II. Title.
    [DNLM: 1. Psychotherapy.   2. Mental Disorders—therapy.   3. Mental Disorders—drug therapy.   4. Clozapine—therapeutic use.   WM 420 D316r   1996]
    RC514.D35   1996
    616.89′1—dc 20
    DNLM/DLC
    for Library of Congress   95-44617

Manufactured in the United States of America. Jason Aronson Inc. offers books and cassettes. For information and catalog write to Jason Aronson Inc., 230 Livingston Street, Northvale, New Jersey 07647.

Preface

Not long ago one of us (K. D.) met Joanne Woodward after a performance of *Arsenic and Old Lace* at the Long Wharf Theater in New Haven. She had acted in many films about people with mental illness, including the *Three Faces of Eve, Sybil,* and *The Glass Menagerie,* and these had made a lasting impression on K. D. As Woodward had given such exceptional performances, two of which were in live theater, K. D. was sure that her gift was partially determined by life experience and a special interest in people whose minds were affected by psychosis. Woodward assured K. D. that she had no particular interest in people with serious mental illness. The characters she played were "just people." And her portrayal of the mad Abby Brewster in Kesselring's (1941) *Arsenic and Old Lace* showed respect and empathy for that character, with no trace of pity.

It behooves clinicians to recognize the humanity of their patients. We are aware that a mentally ill person must be seen first as a person and that her suffering must not be minimized, nor must knowledge of available treatments that may decrease her anguish be neglected. In the 1940s the Brewster family had to be admitted to an asylum. Near the year 2000 we have newer alternatives for people in mental anguish.

In recent years there has been a renaissance in newly developed medications for people with severe mental illnesses. These medications have the potential to improve the most disabling symptoms of psychosis. Clinicians must have a complete knowledge of these medications and their use to be effective.

And yet our book is about the fact that medications, no matter how effective, do not eliminate the need for psychotherapy. Instead, and particularly following years of severe symptoms of psychosis, patients may have a significant need for a psychotherapy relationship through which developmental processes that were previously cut short might occur.

The advent of atypical neuroleptics provides patients with years of severe psychiatric symptoms an opportunity to look at themselves anew. But this new perspective requires significant adjustment. Some patients effectively treated with the new antipsychotic medications seem unable to use their symptom relief effectively. The elimination or significant reduction of symptoms does not always result in global improvement in the person's quality of life.

The absence of disabling symptoms provides an opportunity for a new sense of self to be explored and consolidated. These are processes that occur within interpersonal relationships mediated by knowledge of human psychology, psychopathology, and development—in other words, in psychotherapy. We developed group therapy specifically to address these developmental challenges and the new types of suffering that symptom relief introduced.

The first chapters in this book detail the specific improvements of people who have been afflicted by long-term mental illness. We then describe some of their struggles and our responses to them, which led to the development of the psychotherapy group. Not all visits were made in group treatment. If a patient requested an individual visit or could not benefit from a group session due to discomfort, anxiety, or disorganization, individual contact was provided. We explore some approaches to psychotherapy with people recovering from long-term psychoses and reflect upon the past and future of medication and psychotherapy for these people.

We told the members of our group that we were writing this book and indicated that any of them could refuse to permit us to describe them and that anonymity would be guaranteed. Most of the patients expressed dismay that we would not use their real names in the book. They wanted to be recognized and acknowledged. We have tried to accommodate their wishes through our acknowledgments while still protecting their privacy by concealing their identities in each chapter. We are grateful to all of them for their many contributions.

Appendix D: **Greater Bridgeport Community**
            Mental Health Center
            Information about Clozapine   **221**

References   **229**

Credits   **235**

Index   **237**

Contents

Preface   ix

Acknowledgments   xiii

PART I: AN INTRODUCTION TO CLOZARIL
                  AND PSYCHOTHERAPY IN THE
                  TREATMENT OF SEVERE
                  SCHIZOPHRENIA

1. Watching Clozaril   3

2. Medication Makes People Look Peculiar   15

3. The Impact of Negative Symptoms on the
     Clinician   31

4. Origins of the Feelings Group   43

PART II: THE SIGNIFICANCE OF
           PSYCHOTHERAPY FOR PEOPLE
           SUDDENLY AND UNEXPECTEDLY
           RECOVERING FROM SEVERE,
           LIFELONG, AND DISABLING
           SCHIZOPHRENIA

5.   The Problem of Sanity   57

6.   The Rat Lady of Bridgeport   71

7.   John's American Pie   89

8.   The Mad Italian   105

9.   From Wild Men to Lambs   127

10. Clara's Selves   147

PART III: USEFUL IDEAS AND TECHNIQUES
           FOR PSYCHOTHERAPY WITH
           PEOPLE UNEXPECTEDLY
           RECOVERING FROM SEVERE
           PROLONGED PSYCHOSIS

11. Reflections on Effective Psychotherapy with
     Patients Recovering from Years of Psychosis   161

12. Before, During, and After Clozaril   177

Appendix A: Prescribing Clozaril   193

Appendix B: Greater Bridgeport Community
             Mental Health Center Clozapine
             Protocol   203

Appendix C: Greater Bridgeport Community
             Mental Health Center Clinical
             Management of Reduced White
             Blood Cell Count, Leukopenia,
             and Agranulocytosis   213

DEVELOPMENTS IN CLINICAL PSYCHIATRY

A SERIES OF BOOKS EDITED BY
ANTHONY L. LaBRUZZA, M.D.

The books in this series address various facets of the role of psychiatry in the modern world.

Using DSM-IV: A Clinician's Guide to Psychiatric Diagnosis
  Anthony L. LaBruzza
Filicide: The Murder, Humiliation, Mutilation, Denigration,
  and Abandonment of Children by Parents
  Arnaldo Rascovsky
Return from Madness: Psychotherapy with People Taking the New
Antipsychotic Medications and Emerging from Severe, Lifelong,
and Disabling Schizophrenia
  Kathleen Degen and Ellen Nasper
Chambers of Memory: Vietnam in the Lives of US Combat
Veterans   with PTSD
  H. William Chalsma
Winning Cooperation from Your Child!: A Comprehensive
  Method to Stop Defiant and Aggressive Behavior in Children
  Kenneth Wenning

To my dear mother who gave me life, strength, and courage, and to my precious children, Kurt and Rose, who gave my life a renewed sense of hope, meaning, and purpose.

Kathleen Degen, M.D.

To the memory of Doris and Aaron Nasper, and of Laura Tashman, each of whom lives in me.

Ellen Nasper, Ph.D.

Acknowledgments

Our book is the product of innumerable clinical experiences, conversations, readings, and chance comments that each of us has absorbed through the years. The contributors to our thinking are therefore numbered beyond naming. They include the patients we have treated over the years, our mentors and supervisors, our colleagues, and our friends.

Still, there are specific people who deserve special gratitude for making this book possible. Most of all, we want to thank the patients who gave us inspiration and permission to write about their lives. We would also like to express our appreciation to our colleagues, especially the case managers and clinicians who worked tirelessly with our patients. And our gratitude goes to our friends and colleagues who gave valuable encouragement and suggestions. Our special thanks are extended to Ivan Collazo, Joe Domschine, Sean Gallagher, Tom Harrison, Bobbie Kaltenbach, Ann Marie Kravec, Rosemary Margeson, Larry Phillips, Pamela Ploughman, Vittorio Porcelli, Stanley Possick, William Smiger, Andrea Smith, Dawn Spictzler, Harold Tisdale, Dirk van Donkelaar, and

Mara Zeitz. We thank James Lehane and Steve Atkins for making the group possible and Melissa Garman for her willing ear, warm intelligence, constructive criticism, and support.

Each of us also has benefited from many teachers who have led us to use the best of ourselves as we treat patients. Among these, K. D. would like to thank Edward Hornick, M.D., Irene Labourdette, M.D., James J. Strain, M.D., C. Christian Beels, M.D., Ethel S. Person, M.D., and Oliver Sacks, M.D. who taught me the value of understanding myself and others. E. N. would like to thank David Read Johnson, Ph.D., Charles Gardner, M.D., and Stephen Fleck, M.D., each of whom taught me a bit more about finding my own humanity in my relationships with people with psychoses.

Sandoz Pharmaceuticals and Janssen Pharmaceutica did not sponsor any part of our work. However, thanks are due to Greg Best, Bud Goodwin, and Frank Langone from Sandoz, and to John Bruins and Jim Ryan from Janssen who have graciously provided information and resources that resulted in improved patient care.

Finally, each of us has friends and supporters whose encouragement and enthusiasm kept us going through this project. Among these, E. N. would like to thank her friends Tracy Smith, Sally Stein, Rita McCleary, Tom Landino, and Naomi Shaiken for their confidence in her, and her husband Brooks Barnett, who seems always to have faith and love and tolerance for her when she needs him most. K. D. would like to thank Mona Schneider, M.D., Elise W. Synder, M.D., Charlotte Degen, Carol Choate, and Tom Greenfield for their comments and encouragement.

PART I

An Introduction
to Clozaril and
Psychotherapy
in the Treatment
of Severe
Schizophrenia

PART I

An Introduction
to Clozaril and
Psychotherapy
in the Treatment
of Severe
Schizophrenia

1

Watching Clozaril

> In the midst of his bewilderment, the man in the cocked hat demanded who he was, and what was his name? "God knows," exclaimed he, at his wit's end; "I'm not myself— I'm somebody else—that's me yonder—no—that's somebody else got into my shoes—I was myself last night, but I fell asleep on the mountain, and they've changed my gun, and everything's changed, and I'm changed, and I can't tell what's my name, or who I am!"
>
> Washington Irving, *Rip Van Winkle*

No one was prepared for the effects of the new generation of antipsychotic medications such as Clozaril on human thinking and behavior. Before Clozaril's introduction in 1991, twenty years had passed since any new medications for the treatment of psychosis had been made available for general prescription use. All the standard neuroleptics worked about the same for most people, with differences mainly in their potential side effects.

Clozaril was the first of a new generation of antipsychotics with an improved effect on treatment-resistant or residual symptoms. It was introduced in 1991 for general use in the United States. The sudden improvement in serious persistent psychosis for many people created an awakening. Like Rip Van Winkle, the patients were bewildered and in many ways were reflecting his words, "Everything's changed, and I'm changed, and I can't tell what's my name, or who I am!"

Many patients who awakened needed a change in treatment approach. For some a change in direction of their rehabilitation from grooming and money management to vocational rehabilitation was sufficient. For many people progress did not occur in their rehabilitation despite dramatic symptom resolution. In Part I we describe why we believe there is still a need for skilled psychotherapy for patients taking antipsychotic medications. In Part II we illustrate common issues that arise in psychotherapy with people suddenly recovering from lifelong mental illness and the significance of psychotherapy for particular patients. In Part III we explain the techniques and approaches to psychotherapy that worked best and our expectations for the future.

OVERVIEW OF CLOZARIL'S EFFECTS AND SIDE EFFECTS

The fanfare surrounding the release of Clozaril for general use began before 1991 and centered on two contradictory themes: Clozaril was the drug that could cure or kill people. The first theme was a commonly held belief that Clozaril was a wonder drug with the potential to cure people with severe mental illness. The second theme related to its potentially fatal side effect of bone marrow suppression. The possible bone marrow suppression (in 1 to 2 percent of cases) could leave a recipient with an impaired immune system, making him or her vulnerable to infection. This scared doctors, patients, and families initially, and fear continues to persist, affecting the frequency with-which doctors prescribe Clozaril. Yet, the threat of agranulocytosis has proven to be manageable, similar to the manageablility of agranulocytosis caused by other chemotherapeutic agents (e.g., anti-cancer medication) routinely prescribed for the treatment of severe or advanced physical illness.

Meanwhile, the dramatic benefits of Clozaril, while cited in professional literature, were underemphasized or reduced to reports of scores on the Brief Psychiatric Rating Scale (BPRS).

Many clinicians, however, were aware of the work of Meltzer and colleagues (1990) and other respected psychopharmacologists and knew that Clozaril might reduce psychotic symptoms by 20 to 30 percent over the first six months of treatment in about 30 percent of cases and increase patients' quality of life. Nevertheless, we were not expecting sudden and dramatic symptom relief or the total erasure of ostensible symptoms of schizophrenia.

First generation typical neuroleptics had helped eliminate or reduce the positive symptoms of schizophrenia for many patients. For decades many clinicians considered the positive symptoms (hallucinations, delusions, and thought disorder) to be hallmarks of the illness. Negative symptoms were not recognized as true and treatable, but rather as residual symptoms or "residual" schizophrenia. Conventional neuroleptics do not differ significantly from one another in their ability to relieve positive symptoms. The main distinction between the typical antipsychotics (the only medication that was available for the three decades from 1960 to 1990 for the treatment of schizophrenia) is in the side effect profile. For example, some of the typical antipsychotics are more sedating or more likely to cause movement disorders. However, all the typical antipsychotics have the potential of inducing excessive sedation and disfiguring movement disorders.

Meanwhile, an added disadvantage of conventional neuroleptics is the apparent lack of efficacy for the relief of the negative symptoms of schizophrenia. The negative or deficit symptoms of schizophrenia include apathy, social withdrawal, alogia (poverty of speech), anhedonia (loss of the feeling of pleasure), and loss of initiative. In some cases the typical neuroleptics actually induce a syndrome of negative symptoms ("medication-induced negative symptoms," a feature of parkinsonism), thereby confounding the diagnosis because of the phenomenologic overlap.

Patients who have negative symptoms of schizophrenia or medication-induced negative symptoms are often at a standstill and cannot make progress in their rehabilitation. Negative symptoms prolong hospitalization and require the use of more restrictive outpatient care such as supervised housing and sheltered workshops. Thus, even patients who have a good response to typical neuroleptics are often significantly compromised by their illness.

The complete or nearly complete symptom relief given by Clozaril to people who had been psychotic in the back wards of state mental hospitals for ten to thirty years of their lives, most of whom were ill since adolescence, took us completely by surprise. Similarly, we did not foresee that Clozaril could help the revolving door users of acute care to accomplish control of their positive and negative symptoms outside hospital walls for very long intervals. Meanwhile, other novel antipsychotics became available such as Risperdal (risperidone), described in the literature by Janssen and colleagues (1987) and Marder and Meibach (1994) among others, and olanzapine and ziprasidone, which were available for use only within an approved study; these drugs had the potential to be wonder drugs for some people without the risk of a fatal side effect. There was no recent precedent for the particular transition to recovery people needed to make, nor any automatic provision to provide help. Mental health clinicians were unprepared to shepherd the affected people through this exciting but perplexing and complex transition in their lives. A redesign of treatment was necessary.

THE MIXED BLESSING OF THE DELIVERANCE FROM MADNESS

The new antipsychotics were a mixed blessing to many recovering patients. Writers and observers of the phenomenon of sudden, unanticipated deliverance from severe positive and negative symptoms of schizophrenia have compared the change in patients to an awakening similar to that described by Dr. Oliver Sacks (1974) in his early days of administering dopamine to people suffering from Parkinson's disease. This experience reflects most accurately what we are hearing from people who abruptly improve after ten or more years of their brain malfunctioning due to the mental disease we call schizophrenia. Unlike Rip Van Winkle, patients suffering from severe schizophrenia were conscious during their prerecovery years, but upon awakening, describe their former state as being like "zombies," "I was just a vegetable," or "I felt like a nonhuman." People who suddenly lost their symptoms of mental illness made such statements as "now I can read a page in a book," "I can see street signs," "I can talk to more than one person at a time," "now I don't know who I am," "everything's changed," and "now I have to figure out what I'm going to do with the rest of my life."

Despite unequivocal improvements, sudden symptom relief has turned out to be at least as painful as psychosis for some people. The resumption of a mental life compatible with reality has created many challenges for patients and the clinicians who help them. The reduction in both positive and negative symptoms of schizophrenia, as evidenced by patients' words and behavior and by objective measurements of clinical outcome (BPRS, Global Assessment of Function, Abnormal Involuntary Movement Scale), as well as clinicians' impressions of outcome, was quickly apparent for all patients who accepted a therapeutic course of treatment. A small number of patients could not tolerate the side effects of Clozaril, and either never reached a therapeutic dose or had to discontinue it despite its usefulness. Yet, about 40 to 70 percent of patients who continued Clozaril experienced the dramatic and unexpected alleviation of symptoms that expanded both their capacity for broader psychosocial independence in less restrictive settings and caused an upsurge of other symptoms that we similarly did not foresee. Bewilderment, anxiety, depression, the release of traumatic childhood memories, social phobia, identity crisis, and obsessive-compulsive symptoms interfered with their rehabilitation in currently existing programs.

A twofold change in programming was therefore needed to help them. For those patients who were willing and able to participate in existing rehabilitation groups, the focus shifted from grooming, nutrition, and the development of other independent living skills to vocational rehabilitation and quality of life issues. Additionally, there was a group of significantly recovered patients who were either unable to participate in revised and intensified rehabilitation because their new symptoms inhibited them from successful participation, or they could participate, but achieved below the expected benefit based upon how well their psychotic symptoms were resolving. In other words, Clozaril had delivered them from the jaws of devouring mental illness, suitable rehabilitation was available, and yet they accomplished less than reasonable and expected improvements in their social and vocational lives due to emergent nonpsychotic symptoms. This group of people clearly needed something more to ease them toward a meaningful recovery.

Many of the patients who did not improve in daily life functioning despite an apparent freedom from severe mental illness had complained of symptoms related to the identification and management of intense feelings; the unprovoked retrieval of painful memories such as of child abuse, rape, or an abortion; and a severe identity crisis. Their sense of identity established during adolescence was that of being a mental patient. Those seeking self-understanding required a treatment that had, for the most part, been discarded from programming for those who had drifted downward with advancing mental illness to public sector care. It was also clear that techniques from dynamic and supportive psychotherapy would be critical for this group of Clozaril-treated people to enable them to achieve a significant recovery with increasing social and vocational function.

In response to the need for another treatment approach we began in 1993 a psychotherapy group for recovering patients whom were part of the medication group. We describe the origins and development of the psychotherapy group in subsequent chapters. Here we present the basis for the many thoughts and observations about the compelling and necessary partnership between Clozaril or other novel antipsychotics and psychotherapy.

Our initial psychotherapy group consisted of a nidus of eight members, some with greater needs ("low functioning"), but all with the desire to belong to the group and talk about their feelings. This group of eight remained stable during the first six months. Table 1–1 characterizes the group members by demographics, and Table 1–2 gives their diagnoses. Table 1–3 lists two objective measurements of patient function, the Brief Psychiatric Rating Scale and the Global Assessment of Function, before treatment with Clozaril and after six months of Clozaril exposure.

Although the core group had eight consistent members, other participants were added after six months, and some of the original members left. All of the group members met the eligibility criteria for Clozaril: incompletely remitted schizo-

Table 1–1 Characteristics of Group Participants

Age Range—29–52 average 40
Gender—Three female, five male
Ethnicity—Three African-American, five white
Medical Insurance—Title 19
Duration of illness pre-Clozaril > 10 years

Table 1–2 Diagnosis of Group Participants

Pre-Clozaril:	3 chronic paranoid schizophrenia
	2 chronic undifferentiated schizophrenia
	3 schizo-affective disorder
	(7 of these: substance dependence)
After 6 months of Clozaril treatment:	8 residual schizophrenia (0 of these: substance dependence)

Table 1–3 Objective Measurement of Function of Group Participants

	Pre-Clozaril (N = 8)	After Six Months (N = 8)
Brief Psychiatric Rating Scale	58–36 (47.87 average)	31–20 (25.25 average)
Global Assessment of Function	30 (30 average)	50–80 (57.62 average)

phrenia after two successive trials of neuroleptics—typical antipsychotics such as Haldol (haloperidol), Prolixin (fluphenazine), or Thorazine (chlorpromazine)—for six weeks each; and/or the occurrence of unacceptable side effects to typical antipsychotics. The presence of tardive dyskinesia, tardive dystonia, akathisia, or the tremor of parkinsonian side effects was an automatic indication to offer Clozaril to affected people. Therefore, many of the group members were suffering from some type of movement disorder that drew attention to them and made them stand out anywhere they went as not being normal. Substance abuse or dependence was not a reason to withhold Clozaril. Seven members of the core group were dependent on alcohol and/or cocaine to the extent of warranting a dual diagnosis.

The average and expectable benefits of Clozaril are all or some combination of the following: improved functioning of the part of the brain that controls motion, enabling people to move normally; reduced or resolved positive symptoms of schizophrenia (hallucinations and delusions); reduced aggressivity, length of hospitalization, and cost of inpatient care; improved or resumed family relationships; and improved grooming, social skills, and capacity for involvement in work programs, competitive employment, or return to school. Based upon three years of experience with over eighty patients, to this conventional list we can add without reservation the diminished or discontinued use of alcohol and/or cocaine. We discuss the growing literature to support our assertion of Clozaril's effect on substance abuse in Chapters 8 and 9.

Chapters 2 and 3 provide more information about the physical and psychological challenges to the person with severe and persistent mental illness. We complete Part I with an overview in Chapter 4 of our observations of the Clozaril psychotherapy group (the "Feelings Group") as we watched the unique partnership between Clozaril and supportive/explorative therapy progressively unfold.

In Part II we describe the significance of psychotherapy for some of our patients who, due to new antipsychotic medication, emerged from severe, lifelong, and disabling schizophrenia.

Part III summarizes our observations and understanding of people unexpectedly recovering from severe, prolonged psychosis and the psychotherapeutic techniques we have found useful (Chapter 11). A brief history of the management of schizophrenia and treatment alternatives that are being developed for the future (Chapter 12) concludes Part III.

In the appendices we have included our facility's protocol for prescribing Clozaril and for the clinical management of reduced white blood cell count, leukopenia, and agranulocytosis, as well as information for patients and their family. This material may be useful to other facilities or to clinicians who are initiating a Clozaril Program or Clozaril Clinic.

2

Medicine Makes
People Look Peculiar

Her eyes remained blank, and every gesture was swollen with effort. She spoke now, but softly in a high thin voice and only when prodded gently by Douyon. There was little spontaneous emotion, and when she left the room she walked as if on the bottom of the sea, her body bearing the weight of all the oceans.

Wade Davis, *The Serpent and the Rainbow*

Clinicians who work with the chronically mentally ill become immune to thinking about the ways in which their patients look peculiar. By a poorly understood process that we might call "the six-week phenomenon," after six weeks of continuous contact, clinicians cease to notice the ways in which patients look strange. Unless the symptoms are of recent onset or are worsening, we lose conscious awareness of the client's staring, pacing, foot swinging, shuffling from foot to foot ("the stelazine stomp"), grimacing, chewing, tongue protruding ("fly-catcher tongue"), puckering, twitching, writhing fingers ("piano or guitar fingers"), or walking as if made of wood. The patients rarely complain, and may be unaware of the abnormal involuntary movements even when reminded or asked about them. Yet a novice to the field of treatment of the lifelong mentally ill notices immediately. Remember walking into the waiting room to greet your first client?

How does this insensitivity develop in us? No one knows for certain. Clinicians probably develop a tolerance for the way our clients look peculiar much the way human beings adapt to severe physical pain. After about six weeks of agony, pain perception undergoes a transformation. Although still perceived, the suffering is experienced differently; it is relegated to a different level of awareness.

It does not require a great stretch of the imagination to compare the six-week phenomenon to the transmutation of pain perception when we recall how painful it is to see patients who have lost control of their ability to move. The loss of control is cosmetically disfiguring and often disabling. A tolerance may also develop as we get to know our clients and extend ourselves into a relationship by an identification with the healthier parts of them.

Another theory about why clinicians forget how strange a client looks has to do with how we form and hold impressions of another person. We accept a definition of client that includes the peculiarities of psychosis. Just as in time we adapt to and accept the way a person who has a thought disorder communicates, so we adapt to the abnormal movements as an accepted part of that person's physical presence. Various attributes, no matter how strange, are accepted and are no longer noticed consciously, though readily seen by a new observer.

Tolerance for the patient's appearance may permit a better relationship with the patient. Ignoring the ways in which patients appear peculiar may help them to form and strengthen "neurotic defenses" to assist them in acquiring or maintaining socially valued roles. However, our loss of sensitivity may cause us to lose sight of how greatly patients' lives are affected by looking peculiar. Walking like Pinocchio, unlike the little boy in the story, does not win friends and influence people. Rather, by looking peculiar, a client may become lovable only to a parent or therapist. The impact of peers' rejection, with providers' and family members' acceptance has potential for infantilizing and diminishing a person and fostering dependency.

IS ALL THAT MOVES TD?

Although only infrequently the focus of systematic studies (Yassa et al. 1990), the plethora of abnormal movements that accompany severe mental illness have captured the notice and interest of scholarly clinicians, at least since the time of Kraepelin (1919). Kraepelin was writing about the abnormal movements of people with schizophrenia decades before the availability of neuroleptics like Thorazine (chlorpromazine) or Haldol (haloperidol).

Further confirmation of the development of abnormal involuntary movements independent of neuroleptic treatment is also provided in a recent retrospective study by Turner (1989). This study is based upon a review of asylum case records in England from 1850 to 1889, almost a century before the development of neuroleptics. The author's review shows that over 25 percent of people with schizophrenia exhibited abnormal involuntary movements that would be labeled in the contemporary psychiatric language as tardive dyskinesia (TD). The tardive or delayed-onset dyskinesia that develops independently of neuroleptic medication is called *spontaneous dyskinesia* and is believed to be intrinsic to the schizophrenic process.

According to Casey and Hansen (1984), the prevalence of spontaneous dyskinesia (not medication related) has been reported to be anywhere between 0 percent to 53 percent. Fenton and colleagues (1994) recently studied schizophrenic patients at Chestnut Lodge who had never received treatment with neuroleptic agents up to and including the baseline assessment. In many cases, they found that oral-facial dyskinesias in patients with negative symptoms and intellectual impairment may actually represent spontaneous movement disorders associated with hebephrenic or deficit forms of schizophrenia.

A study by William Glazer and colleagues (1993) investigated the prevalence of tardive dyskinesia among people who have lifelong mental illness and extensive neuroleptic exposures up to 25 years. They found that 68 percent of people with 25 years of exposure to neuroleptic drugs will be afflicted by tardive dyskinesia. Undoubtedly more than 68 percent of people with lifelong mental illness look peculiar if you include all abnormal movements that occur while taking neuroleptic medications.

The people described in these studies would be seen most typically in community mental health centers or state hospitals, although some may still retain enough insurance or family resources to be seen by clinicians in private hospitals and outpatient clinics. If the state system of mental health is privatized (as may soon be the case in Connecticut), clinicians in private practice will be seeing many more people with severe and complicated afflictions, including disorders of movement.

The point of these studies is that spontaneous dyskinesia is inherent in certain cases of schizophrenia and would occur with or without antipsychotic drugs. Yet, although it is well documented that patients having a "schizophrenic body" may have developed spontaneous dyskinesias—that is, schizophrenia-related movement disorders—it is likely that neuroleptic medication plays a contributing role in some of their movement problems. When many patients say that the medication makes them look strange, or their fingers or tongues do not work right, at least some of them are correct. Additionally, clinicians often notice that an adjustment in medication may modify the movement disorder, sometimes for the worse, sometimes for the better.

We cannot distinguish drug-induced from schizophrenia-induced movement disorders. Even if we could, patients who are conscious of their involuntary movements usually attribute them solely to their medication. Therefore, for the sake of simplicity we do not attempt to separate them. Both types of abnormal involuntary movements can be treated. Regardless of their severity, dyskinesias and dystonias can be diminished or avoided, particularly by new neuroleptics, regardless of their source.

THE BIOLOGY OF DYSKINESIA AND THE HISTORY OF ITS RELATIONSHIP TO ANTIPSYCHOTIC MEDICATION

A simple biochemical rationale for the relationship of schizophrenia to involuntary movements is easy to provide. We have known for some time that people with schizophrenia have malfunctioning receptors in their brains. A receptor is similar to a lock (a chemical template) into which a key (the chemical messenger) must fit properly for normal stimulation and inhibition of stimulation to occur. A thought cannot be formed nor a feeling surface without a good fit between the relevant chemical messengers and receptor sites. If too much or too little chemical messenger exists or too many or too few receptors for the messengers are at the receiving end, disorder will result.

For several decades we have suspected that in the schizophrenic brain both dopamine 2 (D_2) and dopamine 1 (D_1) receptors are either too numerous or are being excessively stimulated by extra chemical messengers. All antipsychotic medications until Clozaril were considerably potent D_2

blockers. Until Sandoz Pharmaceuticals developed Clozaril, a weak dopamine blocker, and clinicians observed its extraordinary efficacy for the treatment of previously unrelieved schizophrenia, the role of other neurotransmitters in producing schizophrenic symptoms was not understood. This lack of understanding was reflected in a curious requirement with regard to the development of new antipsychotic medication.

Looking for Cataplexy

Before 1990, in order for a pharmaceutical company to pursue the development of a new treatment for schizophrenia, the Food and Drug Administration (FDA) had to be convinced that the drug could induce cataplexy. Cataplexy is the suppression of movement to the point of collapse. The production of cataplexy was required as evidence of effective D_2 blockade. The equation of a therapeutic effect of medication with the induction of cataplexy rather than with the clearing up of a thought disorder suggests that no one imagined the thinking disorder of mental illness had a life of its own and could therefore be treated separately. The extent to which the agitation of the mentally ill was feared and therefore selected as a target symptom apart from and more important than the thought disorder suggests not only the amount of misunderstanding of mental illness but also the degree to which the mentally ill were dreaded and belittled.

   D_2 receptors do exist throughout the brain and are probably malfunctioning in some cases of schizophrenia. However, there is a high concentration of D_2 receptors in the nigrostriatum. The nigrostriatum (also called the striatum) is integral to movement from our facial muscles to our toes. A D_2 blocker can cause many kinds of abnormal involuntary movements. The type of movement disorder is determined by many factors, among which are exposure to head trauma, drug and alcohol use, predisposing illness such as diabetes mellitus, or genetic polymorphism (differences in individual biochemical constitution).

MORE THAN YOU EVER WANTED TO KNOW ABOUT MOVEMENT DISORDERS

Aware that all that moves is not true tardive dyskinesia, one can now see that matters are even more complicated than first imagined. Yet, another distinction is important to describe.

An accurate description of the characteristics of dysfunctional movement requires placing zebras with zebras and horses with horses (because zebras, though they have similarities with horses, are not horses). A simple method of understanding involuntary movements is to classify them as type A (too much motion) or type B (too little motion). Type A would be the movements of excess, that is, hypermotoric. Type B would be too little motion or hypomotoric. The bad news is that the type A and type B distinction, although compelling because of its simplicity and memorable because of the familiarity to those of us interested in character structure, offers insufficient flexibility to be of real utility. (No one would think rejection of a simple schema would be one of those abhorrent "just becauses." Just because psychiatrists like to mystify what they do?)

Therefore, let us rephrase the issue into a question: What are the differences among tardive dyskinesia, tardive dystonia, tremor (or parkinsonism), akathisia, and acute-onset dyskinesia and dystonia? The conventional answer is that all of the above disorders are considered secondary to neuroleptics. Although we know some of them to be non-neuroleptic-related, or spontaneous, we do not make this distinction in diagnosis because we usually cannot tell them apart. The only clue about which symptoms are due to what cause is derived from a review of the medications.

To better understand the movement disorders, a useful distinction is the categorization of abnormal movements into those with an early or late (tardive) onset and early-onset disorders that persist but are reversible. Acute early-onset drug-induced movement disorders occur within sixty days of beginning treatment. The types include dystonia (a fixation of movement), parkinsonian tremor (four to twelve tremors per second), and akathisia (restlessness). These movements make people look peculiar, but may stop with a reduction or discontinuation of treatment. They often can be relieved by antiparkinsonian drugs such as benztropine (Cogentin), trihexiphenidyl (Artane), or diphenhydramine (Benadryl). But the situation is not so simple. Antiparkinsonian medications have their own side effects. Among them are blurred vision, which can cause squinting. Another side effect of antiparkinsonian medication with anticholinergic activity can be mental confusion, which can cause people to look confused. In our culture, where appearance and first impressions are probably overvalued, others may not be interested in forming relationships with these mental patients.

The acute-onset abnormal movements due to neuroleptic medication usually cause a great deal of distress to those affected by them. However, they usually go away by themselves with or without an antidote. An unknown proportion of cases of acute-onset dystonias, parkinsonism, and akathisia do not go away with treatment and persist over the duration of neuroleptic treatment. Many people with mental illness need continuous treatment with typical neuroleptics in tertiary care centers such as community mental health centers (CMHCs). The CMHCs typically provide care to those with lifelong illness and nearly lifelong neuroleptic exposure. Many people receiving care in CMHCs have acute-onset abnormal movements that become continuous. An educated guess based upon clinical experience is that about half of those treated with neuroleptics have continuous abnormal movements that persist. It is not unusual to encounter patients taking three or more drugs in an attempt to alleviate disorders of movement, thereby creating another cluster of side effects and drug-drug interactions.

In *tardive dyskinesia* slow (less than two per second) choreiform movements occur three or more months after initiating neuroleptics. The writhing movements may affect the mouth, tongue, face, neck, limbs, or trunk. In severe cases the muscles that regulate breathing can be involved (Chiu et al. 1987). If respiration is affected, the patient looks strange because of sighing or gasping without any external cause, and is at risk for respiratory insufficiency. Tardive dyskinesia looks like and may be confused with Huntington's chorea.

Dystonia refers to sustained movements of about five to twenty seconds that can affect fingers, toes, neck, the tongue, arms, or legs. Dystonia can be acute or tardive. Grooming is especially difficult for a person with tardive dystonia. It is not uncommon to see the affected person hold the head while trying to shave, wash, or tie shoelaces. Driving a car or operating other machinery is very dangerous. Tardive dystonia is very difficult to treat, and it usually worsens over time.

Akathisia, from the Greek meaning "not to sit," refers to an inner drive to move continuously, or restlessness. Akathisia may be of acute onset and go away without the need for a continuous antidote. However, in many cases, the akathisia is a persistent side effect of neuroleptic medication that incompletely responds to any treatment. Many patients tell us that this adverse effect of medication is very agonizing. Studies link the presence of akathisia with a higher-than-expected prevalence of suicide attempts and violence. Akathisia is underdiagnosed and the suffering of the patient is often minimized. Shifting weight from foot to foot; purposeful or semipurposeful hand, arm, or leg movements; and an inability to remain lying down or to sleep are other symptoms. The affected person is unable to keep the legs still and has a strong compulsion to pace up and down, feels an inner restlessness, and may appear fidgety. It is hard to imagine that a person affected by drug-induced akathisia would be easy to engage in psychotherapy or that he or she would not be irritated easily.

Parkinsonian tremor consists of about four to six rhythmic involuntary movements per second. The parkinsonian or extrapyramidal tremor is rapid compared to the choreiform movement of tardive dyskinesia. This adverse effect of neuroleptic medication often affects the fingers and looks like pill rolling, but can involve the whole body. Available antidotes may not succeed in reducing this side effect.

Tics, sometimes called tardive Tourette's syndrome, are abrupt irregular movements that can affect the face, neck, limbs, or trunk.

Myoclonic movements are rapid, jerky, and irregular. They are often identified most easily on the face, arms, or legs. If myoclonic movements affect the mouth, tongue, or laryngeal muscles, speech can be impaired. If the legs are involved, falling can occur. Engaging in a reasonable physical fitness program, jogging, swimming, playing tennis or even walking cannot be done. With myoclonic movements, even grocery shopping is difficult.

Bradykinesia is Greek for the suppression or reduction of movement. This is the Pinocchio effect of typical antipsychotics. Bradykinesia is often accompanied by slowed thinking and detachment. A person with bradykinesia initiates movement very slowly. The gait (manner of walking) is slow and unsteady, and the stride is shortened. The gait of a person with bradykinesia is often conspicuous not only for changes in movement of the legs, but also for reduced swinging of the arms. Additionally, the facial expression is diminished or absent (masklike face), and the poverty of thought and speech may be the cognitive representation of bradykinesia. All of these characteristics give a person a wooden or zombielike appearance.

The safety of conventional antipsychotic medications is limited by their extrapyramidal side effects and tardive dyskinesia. The comfort and capacity of patients to perform such needed activities of daily living as bathing, dressing, shopping, doing laundry, and walking are impaired. In addition, the appearance of the affected person is altered, and not for the better. Dating and romantic involvement are difficult if you have abnormal involuntary movements.

MY MOTHER THINKS I'M HANDSOME

The comments provided with the definitions of the abnormal involuntary movements secondary to medication convey some important visual images. Many life long sufferers wear unfashionable, unkempt clothing: shoelaces are improperly tied, heels or toes stick out, buttons are unaligned or closed, clothing doesn't fit (too big or too small), sneakers or sandals and no socks are worn in winter and boots and no socks in summer, the coat is too light or too heavy for the season, there is never an umbrella or raincoat, and the people with schizophrenia smell. The foot may also be shaking or swinging. The psychiatrist often does not know whether the negative symptoms of schizophrenia are not adequately relieved by conventional neuroleptics or the side effects of conventional neuroleptics are responsible for them.

Some of the patients' lack of self-care is caused by progressive schizophrenia, particularly when negative symptoms are present. Conventional neuroleptics do not usually relieve negative symptoms, especially if they have been present for a long time and the neuroleptic may be causing them.

It must be nearly impossible for persons afflicted by abnormal involuntary movements—drug-induced bradykinesia (suppression of motion) or excessive, uncontrolled, unwanted movements—to prepare themselves to look their best, even with excellent motivation. We know that drug-induced deficit symptoms often deplete motivation as well.

Imagine your first job interview. Would you get the

coveted position if your tongue was crossing the plane of your teeth, your jaw was careening up and down and from side to side, and your fingers were moving without a guitar or piano to play?

"My husband was understanding at first," said a woman with schizophrenia who had developed irreversible tardive dyskinesia. She related how she pursued consultation after consultation with prominent psychiatrists and neurologists. Her jaw moved from side to side, and she had uncontrollable grimacing and lip smacking. Her tongue protruded as she tried to form her words. "I feel he doesn't want me anymore. . . . He says he can't love me the way I look." She also described her difficulty caring for her preschool-aged daughter. "I hate to have her see me like this." Her pain was evident, not only from her words but from what she didn't say. Her movements worsened as she spoke. Feeling rejected, facing possible abandonment, and fearful of the future knowing her options for dating and marriage were slim, the patient struggled to maintain her composure.

"Here comes Shaky," said neighborhood people as they ran away or continued a hostile, derisive discourse. These cruel and hurtful words are regularly hurled at one of our tardive dyskinesia patients with the verbal ability to describe these brutal encounters. He regularly attends our Movement Disorder Clinic, desperately seeking help for his TD but finding no relief in conventional treatments. The involvement of his face (perinasal muscles), neck, and shoulders makes his disorder very evident, disabling, and cosmetically gruesome. The Phantom of the Opera would have looked normal compared to this man. He cannot get a date, a seat next to a normal person on a bus, a place next to a person in line in a supermarket, or a kind word. People run from him in fear or make hostile, belittling comments.

Such events are all too familiar in clinical practice with people severely afflicted by mental illness.

For most of the history of the treatment of severe schizophrenia, we clinicians could only notice such events with compassion and help the person adjust to his or her peculiar appearance using various techniques from supportive psychotherapy. We strove to help them obtain some enjoyment from their lives despite their deformities.

Fortunately, movement disorders may be diminishing with the advent of novel antipsychotics such as Clozaril and risperidone. Clozaril may be curative of certain cases of tardive dyskinesia and tardive dystonia. In addition Clozaril does not seem likely to *cause* movement disorders. Risperidone at doses below 6 mg a day also seems to spare people the suffering of abnormal involuntary movements. We do not know whether taking risperidone for many years may cause tardive dyskinesia. Other neuroleptics that relieve the thought disorder of mental illness while avoiding or minimizing effects on motion are currently being developed. Medications in advanced development like olanzapine and ziprasidone offer hope that the future of people with severe mental illness will be better.

In this book, we focus on patients who have suddenly recovered from prolonged schizophrenia while taking Clozaril or risperidone. Some of them recovered also from persistent abnormal involuntary movements that had made them look peculiar. Part of the psychotherapeutic work has focused on their reactions to their new look, and to how they were responding to the changed reaction of other people to their new appearance and behavior.

3

The Impact of Negative Symptoms on the Clinician

> In our secular society, life and death are defined in strictly clinical terms by physicians, with the fate of the spirit being related to the domain of religious specialists who, significantly, have nothing to say about the physical well being of the living. In vodoun society, the physician is also the priest, for the condition of the spirit is as important as—in fact, determines—the physical state of the body.
>
> Wade Davis, *The Serpent and the Rainbow*

In the popular mind, a person with schizophrenia is often imagined as wild, threatening, delusional, and responding to voices only he can hear. In other cultures, people with such symptoms have been seen as spiritually possessed. These flamboyant traits do characterize some people who suffer from schizophrenia, but there are others whose illness presents much more quietly. They are passive, unresponsive, apathetic, usually quiet and undemanding. Psychiatry describes these as the negative symptoms of schizophrenia. Those of us who treat these patients may feel disturbed by their condition, for it can seem that they are devoid of spirit, spiritually robbed or even dead. In our culture the physician is not the priest, even when the problem seems spiritual. In response to people who seem spiritually dead, the clinician may feel in need of skills that are beyond those common to her training. In this chapter, we look at the impact of negative symptoms on the clinicians who treat these patients.

Steve has spent the past twenty years in a psychiatric hospital and was discharged to the community in 1994 (one year before this book was written). Steve's usual physical posture is quite still. He stares off into space, his head tilted up and to one side, his mouth open, eyes fixed, seemingly in a trance. He initiates no communication with anyone and seems barely responsive when others talk to him. With a great deal of encouragement, Steve will engage in an activity, drawing for example. But his activity is entirely solo. He does not relate interpersonally.

At the time of writing he had recently started a new neuroleptic, ziprasidone. The chaplain, who has known Steve for more than ten years, reported that recently Steve raised his hand to volunteer for a day's labor at a Habitat for Humanity Project. She was surprised, but he came along and shoveled dirt diligently during his whole shift. At the end of the day, Steve approached the chaplain, an unusual event on its own. "That was fun," he told her. This was the first report of pleasure she had heard from Steve since she had known him.

Clinicians who work with severely disabled persons with long histories of schizophrenia become familiar with presentations such as Steve's. Steve has many of the negative symptoms of schizophrenia. He is withdrawn, uncommunicative, and unresponsive; takes no initiative; and seems to take no pleasure in anything. Some, but not all, persons who suffer from schizophrenia exhibit negative symptoms. Negative symptoms are thought of as being persistent, underlying, and chronic. They include withdrawal, an absence of emotional responsiveness, loss of will, loss of capacity for pleasure, poor attention, and reduced physical mobility. When interacting with a patient who has severe negative symptoms, it can seem like "nobody's home." Many of us were taught that these symptoms are the hallmarks of chronic disease, with the implication that there is little that can be done for persons whose lives are crippled by them. Indeed, until the advent of the new antipsychotic medications, there was little successful treatment of negative symptoms.

The effect of negative symptoms on people's lives is devastating. In recent years a considerable literature has developed exploring this impact on the patients' quality of life. We look less frequently at the effect of negative symptoms on the clinical staff who treat people who have them. Yet the effect must be profound, for we feel great relief and amazement when patients begin to emerge from years of negative symptoms, when someone "comes home."

DEFINITIONS OF NEGATIVE AND POSITIVE SYMPTOMS

Recent research on the symptoms of schizophrenia describes three "natural dimensions" (Andreasen et al, 1995, p. 341). The positive symptoms are divided into psychotic and disorganized dimensions. The psychotic dimension includes hallucinations and delusions, whereas the disorganized dimension includes disorganized speech and behavior and inappropriate affect (p. 344). The negative dimension includes "affective flattening, alogia, avolition, anhedonia, attentional impairment, and catatonic motor behavior" (p. 343).

Fenton (1995) suggests the need to distinguish between primary and secondary negative symptoms. Primary negative symptoms are intrinsic to schizophrenia and are enduring. They are also called deficit symptoms. Secondary negative symptoms are the result of some other aspect of the illness. They include depression associated with psychosis, demoral-

ization, symptoms secondary to the patient's neuroleptic medication, and symptoms associated with environmental
deprivation.

In clinical practice it can be very hard to ascertain
whether a negative symptom is primary or secondary. It is our
observation that often no efforts are made to draw this distinction because, we assume, clinicians believe there is little they
can do in either case. However, Fenton's (1995) description
makes clear that some secondary negative symptoms may be
treatable through environmental interventions. Indeed, he describes how some treatment interventions may themselves
result in the development of negative symptoms. Some neuroleptic medications, including Clozaril, can induce significant lethargy and sedation. In addition, medication side effects
can include muscular immobility and decreased emotional
responsiveness, which may appear as negative symptoms
(Fenton 1995). The discomfort induced by these secondary
negative symptoms is often cited by patients as a reason to
discontinue medications.

As we have also noted earlier, extended hospitalizations
may contribute to the development of negative symptoms.
Confinement and reduced stimulation can result in decreased
curiosity, drive, and social initiative (Fenton 1995).

Strauss (1989) pushes this discussion further, raising the
hypothesis that negative symptoms function as a form of
psychological self-regulation, a means by which the patient
interacts with his or her disorder. He hypothesizes that "many
of the so-called 'negative symptoms' . . . may reflect a self-
protective mechanism that the person with severe mental
disorder uses to avoid the numerous discouragements and
psychological assaults inflicted by the disorder, by the society,
and even by oneself" (p. 184).

In the past, medications have alleviated the positive but
not the negative symptoms of schizophrenia. We lacked bio-
logically effective treatments of negative symptoms and
sometimes neglected to investigate whether the negative

symptoms seemed intrinsic to the illness or might be secondary to environmental and psychological factors. Thus we may not have done all we could to address some of the deleterious causes and effects of negative symptoms. Indeed, the advent of the new antipsychotics brings negative symptoms into further relief, precisely because these medications permit us to treat them more effectively. This has led us to wonder at our previous inaction and to look at the impact of negative symptoms not only on patients but also on clinicians.

THE IMPACT OF NEGATIVE SYMPTOMS ON CLINICIANS

Positive and negative symptoms have a vastly different impact on clinicians. Patients exhibiting severe delusions may instill anxiety, fear, pity, anguish, or confusion in the clinician. But they can also amuse, delight, and charm us. Many of us find our patients' delusional material quite fascinating, representing extremes of belief that are accessible to our own fantasy lives. We can identify with the belief that we are the king or a famous movie star, because we have been grandiose in our own fantasies. We can identify with the terror of persecutory delusions through our nightmares and anxious fantasies in the awakened state. We are grateful that our cognitive capacity is not so compromised and that we are able to test reality, to recognize our mental contents as internally produced and not representing our actual state in the world. But having known the terror of the nightmare, the anxiety of the daydream, we find within ourselves some elements of experience that support our empathy with our delusional patients.

Hallucinations are perhaps less ubiquitous experiences among clinicians, although many of us have experienced some types of sensory misperception that may have frightened or astonished us. We may not hear voices, but we have internal dialogues, competing points of view, various conceptualizations of our selves with which we communicate. We recognize these mental contents as aspects of ourselves, although at times we find ourselves at the mercy of negative cognitions that make us feel terrible. So the experience of hallucinations may have some measure of continuity with our daily lives.

Thus, through identification, empathy, and probably most important, the intensity of interaction with a patient with severe hallucinations and delusions, we find some avenue for communication. This capacity to abstract meaning from the patient's experience helps us maintain contact with his or her humanity, even when the content itself is clearly not reality based. We can identify with a feeling state or feel compassion for it. We all know several patients whose severe illnesses keep them hospitalized frequently, but who present such powerful emotional presences that we must make a connection to them. The connection may not be pleasant: we may fear, hate, or pity the patient. But we know that a tortured soul inhabits this body, and this knowledge assists us to find ways to help him or her.

It is harder for the clinician to identify with symptoms of disorganization. Word salad and inappropriate affect are harder to place on a continuum with normal experience and are harder to relate to through their affective content, which may be flattened or out of kilter with reality. Our own experiences of mental confusion, if we have had them, were probably frightening. Still, since the behavior of the disorganized person often retains elements of the forms of interpersonal relating and includes affective content, the clinician is able to provide him- or herself with some mental representation that a relationship is occurring.

In contrast, the identification with negative symptoms is accessible, but more powerfully aversive. Most adults have had episodes containing elements of apathy, isolation, and withdrawal, although most of us relate such feelings to episodes of significantly depressed mood. These mental states are particularly problematic for interpersonal relationships; the impact of these feelings on the other is often to feel robbed. Relating to a patient with severe negative symptoms can feel like relating to an interpersonal black hole, where the clinician's vitality is sucked out and no response is returned. Without a response we are left bereft and can experience little efficacy of our presence, words, listening, or interactions. Thus the patient's apathy, isolation, and withdrawal become contagious. So we withdraw and rationalize that the patient does not notice our withdrawal, our rudeness, or our loss of interest.

There is little literature that focuses on the impact of negative symptoms on the clinician. We suspect this is because negative symptoms have historically rendered us so helpless. Clinicians react to negative symptoms, of course, but our reactions are often outside the bounds of what we consider to be a clinical response. Because there is so little that we can do, we experience our ineffectiveness. We are then vulnerable to reacting to people who have severe negative symptoms with irritation and annoyance, anger, indifference, or disgust. These are not prescribed or instructed responses, but they are normal human reactions to frustration and despair. The absence of feedback and response from the patient deprives the clinician of his or her most powerful reward—the sense that the intervention is meaningful and of use to the client.

In addition, patients with negative symptoms often neglect themselves. Their hygiene may be poor, and so they stink. They are withdrawn and apathetic, and so they are often rude, not acknowledging one's efforts on their behalf. They may look like bums, wearing torn, dirty clothing and with rotting teeth. They are indifferent, unengaged, and hard to please. They do not make progress. Clinicians are at risk to interpret these behaviors as laziness, to accuse patients of being dependent and manipulative, to attribute the presentation to character pathology. We feel helpless, and we blame the patient. Several examples of these common reactions illustrate our point. These examples are drawn from our own and our colleagues' clinical experience.

Reacting with Annoyance

A gifted case manager who usually has enormous compassion for his clients yells at a man who seems unable to button his shirt and tie his shoes. The case manager's reaction assumes that the patient's slowness is volitional, rather than reading it as a symptom of the illness. The same case manager would never yell at his patient for responding to auditory hallucinations because he would recognize these as part of the illness.

Reacting with Avoidance

The social worker who exhibits enormous patience with most of her clients finds herself cutting short an assessment with a patient who is minimally verbal. She finds that when she spends time with him she feels empty, purposeless, and helpless. She feels guilty, but knows that she would rather avoid interacting with this patient because there is so little she can do for him. The patient, after all, is stable. No one complains about his unresponsiveness, and since he makes no trouble he is easy to ignore. He is accepted as who he is, and no one entertains hope that he might improve.

Reacting with Neglect

A psychiatrist interviews a patient whose clothing is dirty and who reeks of urine. Although he vaguely observes signs of tardive dyskinesia, he decides not to do a full assessment of involuntary movements during this visit. He tells himself that he can do this assessment at the next visit, hoping that by then the case manager will have gotten the patient to bathe and do laundry.

Reacting with Rudeness

A patient sits in the psychologist's office awaiting an assessment interview. The patient was on time, despite the fact that she was anxious about the meeting. The psychologist's colleague knocks on the door. Rather than saying that she is busy, the psychologist engages in a discussion for fifteen minutes while the patient sits there.

CONCLUSION

We have said some harsh things about clinicians in this chapter, but they are based on observation of ourselves and our colleagues. Indeed, our point is less to criticize the profession for its shortcomings than to explore the reasons we might make some of the decisions that we do. When treating people with severe psychiatric illnesses, we are all confronted by elements of interpersonal behavior that present us with difficulties. Within the psychoanalytic literature these problems are called countertransference, and the concept is quite applicable here. Our patients sometimes look dirty, smell bad, and say things that frighten or offend us. We find aroused in ourselves a mix of feelings that cause us to behave toward our patients in ways that are determined not by what is clinicially indicated, but rather by our internal responses. We can only begin to mediate such behavior when we become aware of our internal reactions and then start to question ourselves.

Those of us who have chosen to work with the severely mentally ill find ways to adapt to these affronts. These adaptations have their good and bad points. In order to be useful to our patients, we must maintain contact with the humanity of the person who dwells within the unpleasant presentation. Our considerable adaptation to unpleasant presentations permits us to do this. It lets us stay engaged and prevents us from shunning the patient. But it may also be a disservice to the patient if we do not ask him to adhere to the expectations of the wider community.

Implicit in our responses are many elements, including our sense of what is possible for this particular person, both in the immediate future and in the long term. We probably ask more of those for whom we have more hope. When we resign ourselves to limited improvement we ask less.

The more interpersonally engaged with us a patient is and the more sense we have of his personhood, the higher we raise our hopes. Thus the symptoms that manifest in withdrawal, apathy, neglect of self, and lack of responsiveness are symptoms that inherently induce less effort from treaters. We feel helpless, and because we feel helpless we tend to withdraw from the patients who induce them.

The new neuroleptics produce startling and profound changes in some patients. These are the best results of treatment. These results also clarify the ways in which our views and expectations of extremely disabled psychiatric patients become limited by the patients' symptoms. We become inured to the extreme limitations our patients exhibit. We are astonished when, as a result of treatment with the new neuroleptics, a much more complete human being is accessible.

4

Origins of the Feelings Group

My experience with the drug is that there is a period when one becomes more lucid and more able to ascertain one's relationship to society. It's like being on a bridge, where one can see clearly where one has come from, and knows the pain one has been through to get to this point has been excruciating and has served no purpose. One must then decide, with the knowledge that one's only area of expertise is as a career mental patient, whether or not to continue the struggle for sanity and increased functioning. The decision is very simply made: if reality is too painful, all one must do to escape is stop the Clozaril.

Linda R. Larson, letter to the editor, The New Yorker

Linda Larson writes compassionately about her own successful experience with Clozaril. She reflects on others' inability to tolerate this success. It was precisely this conflict and the decision to continue or discontinue Clozaril that led us to consider forming a psychotherapy group for Clozaril patients.

Clozaril was first prescribed in our agency in 1991. Initially it was prescribed primarily to patients treated in an intensive case management program who had been unable to maintain stability as outpatients because of poor compliance with medication and treatment. Often the patients did not co-operate with treatment because, in their view, their medications made them sick. We understand this point of view as an expression that the modest relief afforded their symptoms was not worth the discomfort of the side effects produced by their medication.

The intensive case management program provided daily and sometimes twice-daily medication delivery and super-vised self-administration. In addition, a low patient-to-staff ratio permitted clinicians to extend their outreach to assist patients in meeting other daily needs. For example, they took patients to medical appointments, grocery shopping, and family contacts. This program proved highly successful in stabilizing patients, although many continued to exhibit sig-nificant negative symptoms of schizophrenia.

Some patients, however, remained quite actively psy-chotic, despite such attentive case management. Clozaril was initially prescribed for patients who had not derived adequate benefit from traditional neuroleptics. While taking Clozaril, some patients with previously intractable psychoses exhibited marked improvement within several months. Both authors observed this improvement.

We were both struck, however, by the fact that this unequivocal symptomatic improvement presented poignant and puzzling new challenges. One patient in particular illumi-nated the complexities of treatment that arose out of signifi-cant symptomatic improvement. We tell his story to illustrate the process that led us to realize that we needed to provide something more.

ZACK: THE MIXED BLESSING OF SYMPTOM IMPROVEMENT

Zack is a divorced man in his forties who had attended several years of college. He became psychiatrically ill in his twenties, requiring numerous hospitalizations. On traditional neurolep-tics, Zack suffered from severe tardive dyskinesia, and although an attractive, athletically built man he looked unmistakably like a mental patient. Treated with Clozaril, Zack experienced significant symptom remission. He was able to present himself as handsome, articulate, clear thinking, intelligent, and neatly dressed. Off medication, Zack quickly became paranoid and psychotic and looked, in his words, "like a bum." Nonetheless, Zack kept choosing to discontinue his medication. His clinical team was struck by his persistent choice to relapse.

As Zack improved, he became intensely aware of the unfulfilled dreams he had had for his life: to have a career and a family. He wanted to return to professional work. He wanted respect and love from his family, especially from his father. He had difficulty hiding his romantic feelings toward his therapist. He was articulate about his shame, his sense of failure, and the self-loathing stimulated by these unrealized and, he felt, unrealizable fantasies. His father's disappointment in him and criticism of him emerged as the dominant theme in his now clearer thinking. Improvement was inextricably linked to reminders of his lost possibilities and became the opportunity to confirm his failures in his relationship with himself and with his father.

In contrast, Zack's psychosis included a grandiose delusional system in which his "double" was a successful actor in Hollywood. Living in this grandiose fantasy simply required that Zack remain psychotic. His psychosis thus protected him from the huge disappointments of his life. Clarity of thought, in contrast, presented Zack with extremely painful limitations and challenges. In the real world his future was getting shorter, and his current life was barren of accomplishment and intimacy. This contrast seemed simply too awful to bear.

GRIEVING THE CONSEQUENCES OF IMPROVEMENT

Zack's articulateness raised our awareness of his dilemma: improvement brought with it a recognition of his limitations and of all that he had lost. As Larson (1995) describes so beautifully, one realizes that "one's only area of expertise is as a career mental patient" (p. 10). This realization must be especially poignant for those who showed great promise before they became ill, as had Zack, who had realistically dreamed of success in life.

But it seemed likely that Zack was presenting with stark clarity a dilemma that other patients must also be experiencing. When successfully treated with traditional neuroleptics, many of our patients continued to bear the stigmata of chronic illness through negative symptoms (flattened affect, dulled responsiveness, bizarre movement, apathy), whether these stigmata were attributable to the illness or medications. On Clozaril, our patients looked, felt, and were treated in the community as more and more normal. This raised new adjustment challenges from which they had, until this point, been protected.

Zack expressed an impossible ambivalence. When he did well, he had strong wishes for independence. He wanted to reject his identity as a mental patient, to make up for lost time. This renunciation was manifest as a wish to leave his recent past absolutely behind.

HYPOTHESES ABOUT IMPROVEMENT AS A MIXED BLESSING

As we considered the limits of success with Clozaril, the comments made by our patients raised a long list of developmental psychotherapeutic issues. Patients such as Zack, who exhibited significant improvement on Clozaril, now faced the need to adjust to new ways of experiencing the world and the self. These were enormous adaptational challenges that we had not anticipated. On Clozaril many patients experienced significant improvement, particularly the subsiding of negative symptoms. This improvement brought some renewed hope, but hope also brought new possibilities for disappointment. Improved clarity of thought, in addition to enabling increased interpersonal engagement, permitted patients to think about their futures, hopes, and wishes for life that had been deferred due to years of illness. As their symptoms improved, they were faced with developmental issues that were the residue of their lives before the onset of their illness. Among the adjustments demanded we noted the following:

- *Passivity*: The negative symptoms of schizophrenia induce passivity. Loss of the capacity for pleasure, loss of interest, and social withdrawal contribute to this passivity. In addition, adaptation to the institutional demands of mental hospitals also fosters passivity. Passive behavior on the ward is considered compliance; passivity thus earns rewards. If one's own judgment and perception of reality are often questioned (and also unreliable), accepting the ways others define reality may be a useful adaptation. Such passive adaptations, however, do not teach patients to take initiative or to come to know their preferences or opinions. Such self-knowledge is necessary for active engagement. We hypothesized that one task for our patients was to learn to identify and use their renewed functional capacities—their opinions, their preferences, their strengths and weaknesses, their losses, their dreams—to actively take control of their lives.
- *Loss of Social Skills*: Many persons who were chronic mental patients had been removed from their normal social world in late adolescence or early adulthood. The repertoire of social skills that some might have developed before institutionalization suffered from disuse. Many had never developed independent social relationships or fulfilled adult work or social roles. The social skills demanded within the institution might not

match those useful in the community. As people thought more clearly and became more engaged by their social world, these discrepancies became more apparent to them. Improved functioning and awareness thus led to embarrassment and a sense of inadequacy.

- *Mourning Lost Time:* Sudden recovery from years of mental illness confronted some individuals with a vast sense of loss, especially loss of their youth, of opportunities for career development, and opportunities for family. Some had experienced the loss of children, who were removed from their care due to their mental illness. Several had lost a marriage. Most suffered dislocation in their relationships with their families.

- *Disappointments with Family.* Zack vividly illustrates that a person with severe and chronically disabling mental illness may lose the support and love of family and never be able to regain them. Much as they all struggled to remain in contact and involved, Zack's family found it hard to tolerate his slow improvement. They were as disappointed as he in his lost potential, but as a family unit this shared loss caused them to fragment rather than mourn together. This fragmentation occurred in spite of attempts to mend the relationships through family therapy. Zack could not bear the knowledge that he was repeatedly a disappointment to his father, and he constantly sought approval that his father could not give. This wish seemed so centrally motivating to Zack that he could not abandon it to free himself to focus on the pleasure of his own improvement.

- *Adjusting to a Changed Sense of Self:.* Many patients entertained normal fantasies and wishes for their lives before the onset of their illness. Many of them worked hard to renounce those wishes, encouraged by those who treated them, as a "healthy" acceptance of the limits their illness placed upon them. With marked improvement, however, the accepted limitations might no longer be necessary. Who, then, were they? Few patients posed these questions directly, but Zack's repeated refusal to continue with his medication seemed in part an expression of the difficulty in adjusting to a self that now might actually have some of the possibilities he had once had. Perhaps what pained him most was the recognition that his possibilities were foreshortened by his illness. Perhaps he could not bear the possibility that, despite his improved functioning, he might again be disappointed.

For some patients, improvement proved too painful to face. Symptom remission simply provided the opportunity to look at a lifetime of lost possibilities.

RECOVERY FROM MENTAL ILLNESS AS A POST-TRAUMATIC PROCESS

The model of the post-traumatic state (van der Kolk, 1987) may be helpful in conceptualizing some of the difficulties in adjustment to recovery from prolonged severe mental illness. McGorry and colleagues (1991) describe post-traumatic syndromes following recovery from an acute psychotic episode. They note that a single episode of psychosis is highly stressful since it involves extreme anxiety consequent to delusions and perceptual disturbances. In addition, the circumstances of psychiatric hospitalization are often traumatic.

The experience of a prolonged and severe mental illness bears similarities to the experience of severe and prolonged trauma. In addition to the symptoms and situations encountered during the acute phase of illness, prolonged psychiatric illness is an overwhelming and all-encompassing experience. It redefines life, producing profound alterations in one's sense of identity, basic trust in the world (Herman 1992), and confidence in the future. Although the threat is internal, often the experience of mental illness induces a response of intense fear, helplessness, or horror (*DSM-IV*, p. 428). Persons recovering from chronic schizophrenic illness often exhibit features of post-traumatic states, including a significantly altered sense of self and a foreshortened view of the future.

These responses seem to characterize patients resuming more normal functioning on Clozaril after years of psychosis and institutionalization. For most, this was a first experience of clarity of thought in many years, a broadened range of affective responsiveness, and an increased awareness of others. As in a post-traumatic state, this experience required significant adjustment. As with persons in post-traumatic states, the stresses and effort involved in mobilizing to make use of their newfound well-being produced ambivalent responses.

Most of the patients have had little sense of a future. During their illness, their sense of the future was foreshortened by many intermingling events. Their positive symptoms kept them preoccupied and unable to engage in vocational or social development. Negative symptoms caused them to withdraw, disengage, and enjoy little. Even among those who no longer exhibited stark negative symptoms, there was a timidity about exploring the world, a fearfulness that may be attributable to their lack of trust and confidence in their own stability.

Finally, many of our patients had been deprived of the community of relationships that support an individual's belief in his or her own future. Families and friends had often withdrawn. Some families, friends, and patients themselves had been counseled by mental health professionals to relinquish hopes for a family or work life as unrealistic. Within institutions it becomes difficult to imagine persons taking on different, noninstitutional roles. Thus, having aspirations was discouraged by years of institutionalization.

ORIGINS OF THE PSYCHOTHERAPY GROUP

We formed the group with the express intent of helping patients who had significantly improved on Clozaril to adjust to this improvement. Our purpose was to assist them to mourn their lost years and help them reconcile to an identity that did not exclude their experience as a mental patient. It also meant assisting them to articulate and recognize the developmental challenges and conflicts that still needed resolution.

We felt that since the experiences of these massive changes were ones that these patients shared, a group format would be especially useful. We hoped that it would serve to diminish each individual's sense of isolation in struggling with similar issues. We assumed that a group could help each individual member look at the challenges he or she now faced, particularly those of developing friendships, living in the community, establishing a support system, negotiating relationships with family, engaging in meaningful work, and structuring time that was no longer occupied with psychotic preoccupations. We also hoped that a group would validate individuals in grieving the experience of lost time, lost relationships, and lost sense of self consequent to years of disabling mental illness. We hoped that a group of peers might function as a developmental resource for one another, that their shared experiences of problem solving might prove useful to each other. We tried to follow the principles inherent in Lidz and Lidz's (1982) description of the central task in psychotherapeutic work with people with schizophrenia: "The therapist consistently and persistently seeks to foster the patients' latent desires for individuation; and through the therapeutic relationship counters patients' fears of rejection if they assert their own needs or express the hostile side of their feelings" (p. 11).

PART II

The Significance of Psychotherapy for People Suddenly and Unexpectedly Recovering from Severe, Lifelong, and Disabling Schizophrenia

5

The Problem of Sanity

HARPER: Have you ever tried to persuade him that he wasn't Teddy Roosevelt?

ABBY: Oh, no!

MARTHA: He's so happy being Teddy Roosevelt.

ABBY: Once, a long time ago, remember, Martha? We thought if he would be George Washington it might be a change for him.

MARTHA: But he stayed under his bed for days and just wouldn't be anybody.

ABBY: And we'd so much rather he'd be Mr. Roosevelt than nobody.

Joseph Kesselring, *Arsenic and Old Lace*

While Clozaril has been enormously helpful to many people who have had intractable psychoses, sanity is not always what a formerly psychotic person prefers. In this chapter we demonstrate the diverse responses to the alleviation of chronic psychotic symptoms through the contrast between two of our group members, Zack and Paula. Both of these people had suffered years of psychotic illnesses, characterized by unremitting persecutory and grandiose delusions and hallucinations. Both had years of inpatient psychiatric hospitalizations. Both had a significant and dramatic response to Clozaril, when no prior antipsychotic medications had been truly helpful. While taking Clozaril, both Paula and Zack have no evident stigmata of mental illness. Instead, they are intelligent, warm, and articulate adults.

Yet despite this significant improvement on Clozaril, Zack has repeatedly chosen to discontinue his medication while Paula has not. In this chapter we explore their tremendously different reactions to their medication response and its social and psychological consequences. We can only hypothesize about the source of this difference, which probably relates at least in part to the very different early lives that Paula and Zack led.

ZACK

Zack is a 47-year-old separated white male who has suffered disabling schizophrenia since age 16. Before the onset of his illness he was an A student and a superb athlete. During the course of his illness, his symptoms were partially responsive to treatment, and his delusions became pervasive, holding him captive in an exclusive private mental life with resultant social isolation and inattention to personal hygiene.

Compounding the difficulty of his situation was the development of tardive dyskinesia and tardive dystonia that were progressive. He also was affected by neuroleptic induced parkinsonian movements and treatment-resistant akathisia (restlessness). Despite intervals of noncompliance during which Zack would not take neuroleptics, he spent most of his life in psychiatric hospitals.

After taking neuroleptics for most of the past thirty

years, he was jobless, friendless, smelled, and looked, in his words, "like a bum." He was seriously afflicted by abnormal involuntary movements that made him look peculiar and further interfered with socialization and grooming. Zack's only relationships were with staff from the mental health center and with his father. The connections with other family members were weak. They did not want any contact with him because of his past abusiveness, and they limited their communication with Zack to infrequent phone calls.

His father saw him about once a week. During these visits, Zack would occasionally try to do some simple chores such as cleaning the yard or garage at his father's instruction. The effort was usually aborted, ended by his father's belittling comments. Zack's father was unable to discontinue his practice of making frequent derogatory comments. He felt that his son should be doing better given his earlier great potential, and he attributed Zack's difficulties to laziness. Zack's father did recognize that his son had schizophrenia, a mental illness that erodes motivation and the ability to feel pleasure in achievements, and produces cognitive deterioration. However, his understanding of mental illness was also very narrow. Despite many efforts to educate him, Zack's father was unable to extend his understanding of his son's illness to include attributing Zack's passivity and lack of motivation to negative symptoms of schizophrenia that were not responding to conventional treatment.

The outbursts of inexorable criticism and yelling back and forth that occurred when Zack visited his father intensified and became more frequent. The relationship became further strained when his father's infirm wife required more care. The father decided that Zack could not visit anymore as these visits were exhausting for him and he had become afraid of Zack during these outbursts.

During this time, Zack had lived in state-supported supervised housing. He did not have independent living skills and required frequent assistance with money management, grooming, shopping, and preparing meals. He could no longer perform any sports, including such simple ones as ping pong, pool, or bowling, which demanded less skill and cognitive integrity than basketball or track and placed fewer demands upon his social ability.

The outlook for Zack's future in terms of achieving his stated goals of independent living, fulfilling work, and a few close relationships was not good. After thirty years of progressive, disabling schizophrenia, Zack, then 46 years old, was given an opportunity to take a novel medication that had helped others like him beat the odds of a likely bleak future. He accepted the opportunity to take Clozaril as soon as Title 19 medical insurance (Medicaid) agreed to pay for this expensive medicine. Due to the complex medication monitoring system, only five patients were selected as part of the agency's first effort to use Clozaril. Zack was selected without hesitation. The selection criteria included being among the most severely ill patients with an incomplete response to and/or intolerance of side effects of conventional medications. The selected patients also had to want to take Clozaril. We inferred that people who met these criteria were distressed by their symptoms, dissatisfied by their lack of progress in achieving desired goals, and desirous of obtaining better symptom relief. We therefore hoped they would be motivated to comply with the rigorous assessments and weekly blood tests that were part of the Clozaril protocol.

Within two weeks of taking Clozaril, animation came into Zack's face, light came back in his eyes, and his ability to make eye contact returned. There was somebody home! He spoke of an ability to read street signs and to finish a short story he had been reading for a long time. He wondered if he would be able to complete a course at a local college and have his driver's license reinstated. He observed that street traffic had increased substantially since he had last driven a car, and he wasn't sure that he really wanted to drive again. His daily dose of Clozaril had not yet reached the optimal therapeutic dose.

With three months of Clozaril treatment behind him, finally having reached the dose expected to be the minimum effective amount, Zack's appearance, hygiene, and social skills had improved dramatically. No easily detectable movement disorder was evident. Within three months, a sense of humor appeared. He had resumed a relationship with his father and was now allowed to visit his home again for the first time in three years. As time passed, Zack's growing skill at bowling and ping pong gave him a reputation as the only patient who could beat most of the staff. He developed several friendships and took a course at a local college.

Yet, early on Zack's very impressive awakening became complicated. As his awareness of himself and his surroundings free of delusions or hallucinations increased, a different and unexpected distress began to develop. His enthusiasm for school waned as he noticed the youth of the other students in relation to himself and observed their physical advantages and greater success in dating. His academic inferiority was a further source of suffering. He felt unfairly robbed of his youth and its usual opportunities and potential for development. Zack became alternately enraged and despondent. Technological advances overwhelmed him. Simple innovations made possible by computers, such as the conversion of the school library card catalog from index cards in drawers to files stored on hard disks accessible only from computer terminals, made him anxious. Rather than viewing new challenges as an opportunity and accepting available support to learn needed skills and bolster his self-confidence, he felt defeated and refused the outreach rehabilitation resources for the cognitively challenged mentally ill. He declined staff offers of help in mastering these fears. His anxiety increased. His pride was hurt, and he felt belittled by offers of help. No words could reassure him. He could not perform the public speaking expected of him in his speech class, but he experienced staff offers to intervene with his teacher as humiliating. To complicate matters, he became infatuated with his therapist, an attractive but married woman. Shortly after entering a significant recovery from schizophrenia, he told staff that he hated sanity. "Now I have to figure out what to do with the rest of my life," he said with dark humor. In a serious way, however, he spoke of the pain of his newly recovered contact with reality. Like Teddy in *Arsenic and Old Lace*, he preferred to be delusional than be nobody.

Zack in Group

Zack's pain provided the impetus for the psychotherapy group for patients on Clozaril. Staff were aware that for Zack especially, improvement was problematic. We assumed that problems Zack articulated were probably confronting less verbally skilled patients taking Clozaril.

Zack was an original group member, and until he discontinued Clozaril his attendance was quite regular. He was an excellent group member: active, engaged, willing to talk about his own problems, and willing to listen to others. He was compassionate, empathic, and tried to be helpful to other members. The other members were also attuned to Zack's deep sorrow. They actively tried to draw him out about his family conflict and offered him encouragement about his progress. Zack's presence in the group was marked by the relentlessness of his despair. While all of the patients had adjustment problems due to their marked changes in functioning, none seemed as hopeless about the future as did Zack (an irony, given Zack's far greater potential than many of the other members).

Zack discontinued Clozaril after one year of improvement because "I want to be crazy.... That's the only life I've known for years." A compelling delusion that dominated his thinking was about his double who worked in Hollywood making financially successful films. The delusion was a mixed blessing. His double was keeping all the earnings. According to Zack, a portion of the double's profits was his. Someday, the double would be forced to pay Zack royalties to make up his full share of the profits. This and other delusions protected Zack from intense unwanted feelings, such as grieving the loss of his youth. They also helped him avoid increased expectations of himself that he and others held. Additionally, his retreat from sanity released him from the painful task of planning a future without the potential for high achievement that his youth had given him. Zack was unable to trust that the mental health system and he could form a partnership that could help him design and accomplish a future that he would want.

Zack's recovery and return to madness followed a checkered course. After months of active schizophrenia, he again asked for Clozaril. He wanted to experience life again free of mental illness so he could improve his connection with his family, have a close relationship with a woman, and get a job. He thought that Clozaril could help him. He went back and forth between Clozaril and typical neuroleptics, never resolving his ambivalence. Zack's wish to be free of mental illness was reminiscent of the fabled town of Brigadoon. According to the story by Alan Jay Lerner as told by Bordman (1978), the village minister was troubled by encroaching outside influences so he went to a hill beyond the town:

> There in the hush of a sleepin' world, he asked God that night to make Brigadoon an' all the people in it vanish into the Highland mist, jus' as it was for one day every hundred years. The people would go on leadin' their customary lives; but each day when they awakened it would be a hundred years later. An' when we awoke the next day, it was a hundred years later. [p. 557]

Like the minister in Brigadoon, Zack wanted an awakening that occurred only now and then and under controlled circumstances, timed to his level of comfort. Like the village minister, Zack sought to avoid threatening experiences that were painful to him. He lacked the confidence that he could master these perilous experiences, and he was drawn toward dissolving his sanity, much like the town that, after 24 hours, vanished into the Highland mist.

PAULA

Paula is a 39-year-old single black woman. Her family was working class, her father harsh and abusive, and her mother alcoholic. Paula's own alcoholism began at age 12, and her life has been rife with major interpersonal and environmental stress. She is HIV positive and has known this for the past nine years.

Paula is, by any measure, a Clozaril success. Her massive volumes of medical records attest to over fifteen years of treatment during which Paula was paranoid, angry, threatening, aggressive, and generally unpleasant. She was chronically delusional and severely alcoholic. Since taking Clozaril, Paula has changed markedly. She is usually reasonable, quiet, warm, and concerned about other people. She is rarely angry and then appropriately. Her thought processes are clear, and she exhibits no delusional material.

History

Paula was the third of four children. She was born in Louisiana and raised in Bridgeport, Connecticut. Paula's father is alive, as are her older brother and sister. Her younger sister was murdered in 1984. Paula's mother died at age 43 when Paula was about 12. The immediate cause of death was cardiac arrest, but Paula's mother had been a heavy drinker and Paula says that her mother died from drinking. Paula's older brother also has an extensive psychiatric history and has been diagnosed with paranoid schizophrenia.

Paula's psychiatric history started in 1976, at age 17, when she was admitted for alcohol detoxification. By her own report, Paula started drinking at age 12. She drank heavily after age 15, and by age 17 she was frequently publicly drunk. She had many hospitalizations for alcohol detoxification and depression during her late teens and early twenties. She made documented suicide attempts at ages 15, 18, and 19 by jumping out of windows. Her medical record describes knife wounds, blunt trauma, and razor blade scars as consequences of her suicide attempts and gestures.

At 18, Paula reported having been "raped by eight men in Greensboro." Records describe her as frightened and depressed, becoming "vacant" and staring. At age 19 Paula described having "feelings of strangeness," being isolative and angry and wishing she was dead. Records indicate that at age 26 Paula was struggling with issues of alcohol and "sexuality" (sexual orientation) and was referred to an incest group. (Neither her sexual orientation nor a history of incest has emerged as issues in the psychotherapy group, but Paula has made clear her wariness of intimate relationships with men.) At age 28, Paula was living with a boyfriend who was beating her and forcing her to prostitute herself.

Throughout the 1980s, Paula continued to have frequent psychiatric and alcohol detoxification admissions, although she often discharged herself against medical advice. Her follow-up with outpatient treatment was poor. Paula carried many diagnoses: Alcoholism, Bipolar Disorder, Dysphoric Reaction, Borderline Personality Disorder, and Schizoaffective Disorder. These diagnoses captured Paula's depression, mistrust, rage, and disorganization. She was medicated with neuroleptics, antidepressants, and antianxiety medications. By the mid-1980s, Paula was described as having paranoid and grandiose delusions, specifically that she was having a child by God.

Paula in Group

Paula has been a member of the Clozaril group from its inception. Her behavior within the group has changed more markedly than that of any other member. When she was first discharged from the state hospital, Paula was someone to avoid. She would stand glowering in the hallways waiting for her case managers. She was angry, hostile, and paranoid, and it took virtually nothing to provoke her. In the group Paula was angry, frequently storming out of the room after unintentional and minor slights. She interpreted minor comments as put-downs and found interaction threatening and intrusive.

During a group session early in 1993, Paula interpreted a benign comment to her as derogatory. On the surface, she was angry and ready to storm out. We inquired, however, about her anger. Might she be hurt as well? Paula found this inter-pretation accurate, felt relief and gratitude, and was willing to discuss her hurt. Her response suggested that her hurts were rarely recognized or validated by others or at least that she had difficulty internalizing that recognition. She was able to agree that an angry response protected her from hurts that others might not care that they had inflicted on her. Paula began to manifest some distance from her paranoia and was able to articulate the sequence of events by which her experience of a slight became another's intention to hurt her. However, in spite of how strongly interpersonally related she was, Paula asserted that she preferred not to need people.

Paula was the most articulate of the women in the group. She often protested that she felt uncomfortable as the focus of attention, but equally often, she spoke up to take the floor. Indeed in the first few months of the psychotherapy group, Paula focused largely on her conflicts about attachment to others.

When the group resumed in September 1993 after an August break, Paula vehemently denied that she had missed anyone in the group. During that same meeting Zack announced that his divorce had been finalized. He expressed relief that a burden had been lifted, but Paula noticed that he also seemed sad. They talked for a time about Zack's sadness and his relationship with his ex-wife. Thus empathy and concern for others emerged.

Paula stabilized significantly with Clozaril, exhibiting what seemed to be an optimal response. She is better, apparently in all ways. She has not seemed conflicted about her improvement and seems to be accepting of her life. She grieves her chronic illness, but does not exhibit what one might consider the residual developmental lag. Characterologically, Paula exhibits some obsessional features: she is meticulous in her appearance and keeps her apartment extremely clean. She exhibits strong moral and moralistic beliefs about behavior and seems to act according to her beliefs. She abuses no substances and seems to experience no temptation. She has not had a drink since shortly after her diagnosis as HIV-positive.

Paula does not evidence distress about her significant improvement. We speculate that this major change has been more tolerable for Paula than for Zack because it presents her with less internal conflict, which may be due to her extremely stressful childhood. There was little from her early life that suggested to Paula that adulthood would bring accomplishment, satisfaction, security, or success. Perhaps for this reason, there is less for Paula to reflect against for a sense of disappointment and loss. Paula seems to be able to take pleasure in her recovery and to enjoy her current life with much less regret about time lost or opportunities missed.

After three years, Paula developed medical problems that required her to discontinue Clozaril. She was switched to risperidone, with continued excellent results. Her participation in the Clozaril group (she suggests we change the now-inaccurate name) continues to be active and if anything to grow in depth. She often shares the leader's role of questioning, listening, and trying to help others explore their experience. Paula is remarkably compassionate, constructive, and self-reflective. She speaks little of her chronic physical illness, but has had recent episodes of depression that may be related to her slowly worsening medical condition.

In this chapter we described two patients from our group who shared a very positive symptom response to Clozaril—it worked—but who differed strongly in their reaction to that response. For Zack, the pain of improvement and the issues he had to face proved too much to bear. For Paula, the relief from madness is welcome, and she relishes her improved functioning. We can only hypothesize about the reasons for these strikingly different responses. Part of the explanation is probably in the vastly different expectations they had of their lives: the fact that Zack might have hoped to achieve so much more makes his grief in his illness that much harder to bear. Paula, in contrast, was offered very little by her fates. Although she claims that childhood was satisfying and fun, the record of her life from adolescence on speaks of disappointment and deprivation. We share joy in Paula's recovery, even in its poignant context of her potentially fatal illness. And we grieve for Zack that we cannot help him enough to make sanity bearable.

6

The Rat Lady of Bridgeport

I got the kind of madness Socrates talked about,
"A divine release of the soul from the yoke of
custom and convention." I refuse to be intimidated by
reality anymore.

After all, what is reality anyway? Nothin' but a
collective hunch. My space chums think reality was once a
primitive method of
crowd control that got out of hand.
In my view, it's absurdity dressed up
in a three-piece business suit.

I made some studies, and
reality is the leading cause of stress amongst those in
touch with it. I can take it in small doses, but as a lifestyle
I found it too confining.
It was just too needful;
it expected me to be there for it all the time, and with all
I have to do—
I had to let something go.
       Jane Wagner, *The Search for Signs of Intelligent Life in the*
                                                    Universe

As part of the second wave of deinstitutionalization from state hospitals, people with persistent mental illness were offered vigorous rehabilitation and support services in the community to help them adjust to life in a more natural environment. The effort to downsize state hospitals began in the early 1980s and gradually became the objective of state departments of mental health all over the United States. One result of this downsizing was the treatment of formerly life-long institutionalized, severely mentally disabled people and high users of acute psychiatric care (revolving door patients) in places visible throughout the community and in many social contexts. Those people with major afflictions who were formerly hidden on back wards or caught in an endless turnstile that continuously moved them in and out of the hospital thus achieved high visibility.

This effort to treat the seriously mentally ill in the most natural environment (1984–present) differed from the first wave of deinstitutionalization (1970s). A great deal had been learned from the shortcomings of the methods that were used in the first wave of downsizing. Also, more had been discovered about the severity and tenacity of residual (or negative) symptoms of schizophrenia. The concept of negative or deficit symptoms of schizophrenia was beginning to find its way into the psychiatric literature. The awesome resistance of negative symptoms of schizophrenia to conventional treatments was slowly dawning on clinicians. Early discharge from the hospital with easy access to medication but no supportive services or outreach may have prevented the occurrence of social deficits caused by excessive institutionalization as described by Erving Goffman (1961), but failed to provide for those people whose negative symptoms of schizophrenia eroded their motivation, cognition, capacity to feel pleasure, and self-reward systems. Becoming chronic often meant that positive symptoms such as hallucinations or delusions were adequately relieved by typical antipsychotic medication, but negative symptoms persisted. Ironically, though presenting an enormous obstacle to significant rehabilitation, negative symptoms were usually attributed to laziness, dependency, or passivity or else were ignored.

The most effective measure to help people avoid rehospitalization and achieve stability in their community was intensive case management (Degen et al. 1990). This treatment modality offered rehabilitation and provided help for needed daily activities such as bathing, money management, cooking, and doing laundry in supervised settings. The hope was that the rehabilitation would be internalized, thereby enabling future maximum optimum independence. In other words, a recipient would be able to case manage him- or herself at some future time. The goal was to create a safe place for mentally challenged people, with treatment tailored to fit the individual and offering the least restrictions possible somewhere between the asylums and the streets.

THE ROLE OF PSYCHOTHERAPY IN A CASE-MANAGED WORLD BETWEEN THE ASYLUMS AND THE STREETS

By the mid-1980s the provision of conventional psychotherapy for people who could not get out of bed, bathe, get dressed, prepare meals, manage their own money, or keep medical appointments on their own recognizance had diminished. The focus of treatment was on case management and rehabilitation. Psychotherapy was offered to very few people with severe negative symptoms of schizophrenia in community mental health centers.

The elimination of typical psychotherapy made sense economically as well as therapeutically. Traditional psychotherapy had little chance of efficacy for the treatment of inveterate negative symptoms of schizophrenia. With its office-based, one staff to one patient requirement, and twenty- to sixty-minute time commitment, conventional psychotherapy was very expensive. The unfavorable cost-effectiveness profile of conventional psychotherapy led to its abandonment as a treatment of choice.

With the advent of novel antipsychotics, relief of negative and positive symptoms of schizophrenia created a new need for psychotherapy. The sudden reduction in pervasive, persistent delusions and hallucinations and the recovery of motivation, energy, volition, and the ability to experience pleasure from something other than cigarettes were a mixed blessing. Patients were relieved of terrible suffering, but were left with new problems. Having recovered skills to take care of themselves, they no longer needed conventional case management, but became stuck in a plethora of newly awakened problems. They were in need of some relationship-mediated psychotherapy at a time when the availability of psychotherapy had lessened.

REALITY IS STRESSFUL FOR THOSE IN TOUCH WITH IT

Trudy, the shopping bag lady in Jane Wagner's play (1986), epitomizes the struggle of many people with severe schizophrenia who view sanity with mixed feelings. Trudy has florid symptoms of psychosis, and she has not entered a significant recovery from her symptoms. Yet she has retained her eloquence and recounts her many objections to reality. She thinks reality is too intimidating and confining. At a late point in the play she says,

> But I don't ever want to sound negative about going crazy.
> I don't want to overromanticize it either, but frankly,
> goin' crazy was the best thing ever happened to me.

> I don't say it's for everybody;
> some people couldn't cope. [p. 17]

For Trudy, the benefits of madness outweigh the disadvantages. However, craziness, as she calls it, is also fraught with difficulties, and some people would not be able to handle the agonies of madness.

Indeed, most of our patients, before recovering from serious persistent schizophrenia, were not able to articulate as well as Trudy their feelings about being mad and being sane. However, later in their recovery, as Clozaril began to take effect and they retrieved cognitive skills and psychosocial competence, patients were able to tell us of their own struggles as reality, both exterior and interior, was suddenly forced upon them without much preparation or guidance.

THE STORY OF MARY

Mary typifies the ambivalence many patients feel toward significant and sudden recovery from lifelong mental illness.

Mary was always special to the staff at our inner-city community mental health center. Despite having active symptoms of schizophrenia that were poorly controlled by conventional antipsychotics, she retained fragments of psychosocial capacity that seemed to have splintered off from the disease that was inexorably eroding her mind. Her sense of humor and compassion for others were held captive under a hermetic seal. These qualities would surface when least expected, sometimes in the throes of a terrible crisis. Attempts at psychotherapy ended, however, after about ten years of being mentally ill, as her symptoms progressed and she spent much of her time in a disorganized frame of mind, with an unsatisfactory response to conventional neuroleptics. She was unable to care for herself, so that her most permanent residence became the state hospital. Her family was uninterested in spending time with her—she had become a burden. After twelve years of severe illness, having used up vital resources, she was no longer able to afford private psychiatric care.

There was nothing remarkable in Mary's description of her life before developing mental illness. Her history according to medical records was in concert with her memory of achieving such developmental milestones as walking, talking, completing toilet training, and attending her first days at school, like many other children who would not go on to develop severe mental illness. In Mary's opinion, when she was 8 years old her normal development ended when she gained a lot of weight. Then "I lost my self-esteem" and "have not gotten it back." She recalls being teased continuously by her peers. She had very little social life as an adolescent because of the weight problem and because she never really broke away from her family. She blamed this inability to separate to some extent on her religious upbringing.

Mary became sexually active with a partner at the age of 21. Her first experience resulted in the conception of her son. His birth seemed to change her. She began to hear voices shortly after he was born. She did not marry her son's father and had very little to do with him. Within ten years after the origin of schizophrenia she no longer had any friends.

She had achieved good grades in school (A's and B's) and graduated from business school with honors. Her father was an alcoholic and had little to do with the family. She was very close to her mother who had a major role in raising her son.

Her drug abuse began at age 17, well before the birth of her son and before her first psychotic episode; it began with beer and a few barbiturates a day. The alcohol problem increased. She was eventually consuming four quarts of beer a day with many barbiturates. She also took LSD once, which resulted in a bad trip. Her dependence on alcohol and barbiturates ended at age 21. The reason is unclear and may be related to her becoming disorganized and thereby incapable of obtaining drugs. She experienced blackouts and visual hallucinations of bugs and snakes.

Her older brother was able to fulfill his earlier academic promise and became a successful engineer with a stable marriage and children. In contrast, her self-description was "I was always fat, ugly, and just got uglier." Many suicide attempts checkered her life as a mental patient. Attempts to take her life were often precipitated by voices telling her to kill herself. Mary often took pills, cut her wrists, or did both. She felt convinced that she was an anti-Christ and was going to destroy the world by fire. Although she was able to work for five years as a secretary after completing business school, as her illness advanced, she was afflicted by the belief that the word processor she used at work was talking to her. This experience was frightening and humiliating. Her boss, who was initially sympathetic and concerned, complained that Mary was not taking any interest in her work. He eventually became impatient with her after months when she did not improve, and he fired her. After twelve years of illness, with a lessening ability to hold a job for more than three months, at the age of 33 she gave up and refused to try to work again.

Psychotherapy, though modified for a person with pervasive, persistent schizophrenia, had no impact on her deterioration. After reaching the conclusion that psychotherapy raised hopes and expectations that set the stage for failure, the outpatient therapist referred her to a new program that provided supervised housing, help with entitlements, and general support for other vital and basic activities of daily living. The Assertive Community Treatment Program (ACTP) offered only intensive case management, which was a continuous, hands-on form of rehabilitation in which Mary at first was only able to be a passive participant, utilizing only psychiatric evaluation alone and medication monitoring by trained staff. Mary's aptitude for participating in healing psychotherapy had been erased by severe, advanced mental illness. Deterioration advanced despite the very best attempts at state-of-the-art medication and psychotherapy.

Outcome of Innovative Programming

Some improvements occurred during Mary's treatment in the novel pilot program, the Assertive Community Treatment Program. There were several years of passive compliance, that is, going along with treatment plans made for her; for example, going to the supermarket with her case manager to buy groceries from a list mostly prepared by the case manager. These activities of daily living required constant guidance and reminders in her supervised housing. After a few years of intensive supervision, Mary regained the capacity to carry out some activities of daily living on her own initiative. Mary's sense of humor and sensitivity to the feelings and predicaments of others returned. Her hospital admissions were reduced from two long ones each year to two week-long hospitalizations every two years. She took her medication with little prompting after the first six months in the program. She was able to manage her grooming, money, and housing (supervised) with some assistance outside the structure of a hospital. Eventually she was able to live in her own apartment with daily visits from staff who brought her medication, observed her self-medication, and assisted her in a less intensive way with grooming, money management, nutrition, and other vital activities of daily living.

There were no further suicide attempts. She accepted voluntary admission to the hospital when she became sexually preoccupied, heard voices telling her that she was going to die soon, or became fixated on the rats she believed were infesting her apartment. Though she was convinced of her impending death and spoke openly of the probable date of her demise, she claimed that this conviction did not upset her since she was ready to go into an afterlife. Yet there was no active plan to expedite her death.

She was unable to work during this time, however. Mary felt that her poor ability to concentrate, learn new things, function under stress, or take any spontaneous interest in her life would interfere with her efforts and result in her being fired, thus repeating past failures. She remembered her former job as a secretary in a travel agency as very stressful, with a great deal of pressure to work rapidly. Nothing and no one could convince her to try working in a sheltered workshop. She developed extensive somatic preoccupations with her feet, chest, and bowels. When her doctor-shopping and repetitive exposure to invasive procedures failed to reveal any organic problem, she insisted that it was clear the doctors had simply missed the diagnosis.

Her painful feet often became the reason to stay in her apartment, where she said she was tortured by rats that ostensibly were everywhere, keeping her awake all night with their noise. Additionally, she believed that the rats might make a meal of her, and she frequently pointed to areas of her body that she believed showed rat bites.

The staff were dubious that Mary could get any better since she seemed to derive primary and secondary gain from her rat delusion and physical problems. The rats may have satisfied some inner need to see herself imprisoned and persecuted by some feared creature as a punishment for imagined wrongdoing. By tormenting her, the bad rats may have relieved guilt and self-criticism, thereby making her life more bearable. Staying in her apartment with her rats (she could not leave due to the poor physical health she imagined she was afflicted with) relieved her dread of having worse persecutory ideas that may have been precipitated by leaving a familiar place. It was not clear to what extent Mary was truly a treatment-refractory schizophrenic who only obtained partial relief of symptoms from standard neuroleptics and adjuvant medications. It was clear that she had significant psychological aspects to her illness that helped her avoid other less wanted stressors. The emotional facets of Mary's illness were impervious to many attempts to provide psychotherapy, and her delusions seemed to be getting more intricate and pervasive.

Taking a Wonder Drug That Can Kill People

Expensive miracle medication with a potential to cause death is generally offered only to a small number of carefully selected patients. Ordinarily, the criteria for consideration include not only an incomplete response to conventional medication but also a strong motivation to improve and the ability to understand and cooperate fully with needed aspects of treatment. Because of the potential for Clozaril to suppress bone marrow production of white blood cells, a weekly blood draw for a white blood cell count is a requirement, possibly for the entire duration of treatment. The white blood cells are a necessary part of our immune system; a person who did not have adequate white blood cells would surely die of an uncontrollable infection. There was no way of getting around the weekly blood draw. In order to have an opportunity to take the wonder drug Clozaril, which had helped so many other people with similar treatment-resistant psychotic symptoms, Mary would have to have a weekly blood sample drawn by puncture of a vein. In addition to Mary's dislike of anything new and unfamiliar and her attachment to familiar yet agonizing symptoms, she hated and steadfastly avoided needles.

Mary's various reasons for not taking Clozaril delayed her treatment with it for two years. After more hospitalizations and clearly worsening symptoms, she finally agreed to all the treatment requirements.

Mary's Rat Poison

Treatment with Clozaril did not get rid of her rats quickly. That delusion was the last to disappear. "They're gone," she

cheerfully announced one day. "I don't see them anymore
either. . . . You know, I used to see them, too. . . . Maybe I
didn't tell you. I knew you would think I was crazy. But they
were really there." It was several years before Mary began to
realize that the rats were delusional, a symptom of mental
illness that was relieved by better medication.

After initial treatment, the obvious and foreseeable
events occurred. Mary did not require any further hospitalizations or intervals of intensive supervised housing. Her capacity to initiate normal activities of daily living without
continuous staff support returned. Her self-esteem and sense
of humor became stronger, and her joking developed certain
refinements. "You should have told me Clozaril can get rid of
rats! I would have taken it sooner," she commented.

The best change of all in Mary was totally unexpected
and unforeseeable. Within a year of beginning Clozaril,
Mary's emotional lability had diminished appreciably and her
cognitive capacity had improved to the extent that she was
now able to engage in relationship-mediated expressive psychotherapy.

Yearning for a Relationship/Fear of a Relationship

Mary had recaptured sufficient cognitive and affective ability
through the adequate relief of her psychotic symptoms to
enable her to participate in expressive psychotherapy. At this
point in time, however, psychotherapy was no longer routinely available in community mental health centers. It was
therefore necessary to make use of what services we had
readily available, especially case management and the relationships with the case managers. It was also necessary to understand whether expressive psychotherapy would have
anything to offer her beyond her customary treatment, which
we were trying to tailor to her unique situation. Since she had
suddenly awakened from severe mental illness, she had fewer

problems with psychosis, but a plethora of other problems quickly surfaced. Her relationships with case managers and the use of psychoactive medication to control emergent anxiety and depression had little impact on these problems. It became impossible to discern whether drug-drug interactions were enhancing her symptoms or whether her nonpsychotic but nonetheless painful symptoms were worsening. Mary was able to speak of terrible loneliness, of feeling inadequate to meet societal demands, of confusion about what was real and what was illusory, and of worry about money and paying bills, how she looked, and how to make friends. Who she was filled her with dread. She became very agitated and increasingly complained about physical symptoms that seemed to have no organic basis. She refused to do things that she was clearly capable of, like walking to the mental health center for her treatment or taking public transportation, going grocery shopping by herself, and managing her leisure time in a constructive way. She failed to derive pleasure from anything.

She struggled with an intense longing for a close relationship with her son, brother, mother, or with a new acquaintance. However, her yearning was not fullfillable as she was overwhelmed by fear and avoided people. Work was impossible since she found sheltered workshops beneath her, but feared that she would mess up as she had done before at a real job and would be unable to stop criticizing herself for her repeated failures.

Mary was stuck at an impasse, filled with intense desires for a normal life, with an apparent ability to learn the needed skills, but unable to move forward for reasons stemming from her emotional and mental life. A simple way of viewing Mary's conundrum was that she had been transformed too quickly from a severely ill mental patient to a person who looked and acted normal. But she lacked a grasp of this intense change in terms of an evolving self-definition, mood regulation, and development of a future orientation. She was unable to make a plan or participate in making a plan for achieving

desired goals and had the appearance of being her own worst
enemy. She began to demand more and more pills to buffer
painful symptoms.

Desperately Seeking Psychotherapy

Unanticipated suffering overtook Mary as it had other people
suddenly recovering from severe mental illness by virtue of
wonder drugs such as Clozaril, risperidone, or other promising antipsychotic medications that are undergoing development and are approved for use in a study. Their agony was
largely unresponsive to the prevailing treatments that were
routinely available. Psychotherapy, either group or individual, was not simply a measure of last resort, but a logical step
considering the tenacity of anxiety and dysphoria that was
based not on psychosis or chemical imbalance but rather on
accelerated recovery.

THE DIRECTION OF PSYCHOTHERAPY

Psychotherapy had the difficult task of helping Mary and
others with their unique suffering. Lifelong severe schizophrenia had robbed them of vital experiences that might have
helped mold internal capacities to react to the sudden retrieval
of cognition, memory, and realistic perceptions. The sudden
recovery from prolonged and pervasive mental illness called
upon affected people to use approaches and skills that they
never had the opportunity to develop.

   We were struck by the extent to which Mary's identity
was based almost completely upon being a mental patient.
When she no longer could experience herself entirely in this
way and was startled to notice that others no longer reacted to
her as if she was mad, she was stuck. She spoke of feeling anxious, confused, and empty. In addition, there was a problem of
trusting herself. How could she trust which impressions were
real and which were delusional? When she felt too much pres-

sure upon her to socialize and date, she commented that she could not. "How can I? Before I took Clozaril, whenever I lost my glasses, I used to be sure that someone came into my apartment and took them. Now I know no one came in and took my glasses. So, where did they go? Until I can figure out where my glasses went, I am not ready to go on a date." Many such personal reflections made us aware of other critical problems Mary was having. Both the difficulty learning to distinguish reality from fantasy and trusting her ability to make this important distinction were troubling her and consumed a great deal of energy. Her lack of self-confidence about matters that normal people sorted out automatically was intimidating and humiliating to her. She was unaware of the normal experience of misplacing or losing things. It surprised her to hear that all people misplace things from time to time. She did not react to the explanation that most people sometimes forget where they have put important things. Until the concepts of what is normal were internalized, it was impossible to urge her to consider that maybe the misplaced article may have had some symbolic meaning and been lost for some unconscious reason. We certainly withdrew pressure upon her to rapidly increase socialization or begin dating.

Constructing a broader sense of identity, distinguishing reality from her private mental life, learning to trust her discernment, identifying feelings, regulating intense feelings, setting reasonable and ego-compatible goals, and achieving a socially and personally valued role in society were the major objectives of psychotherapy for Mary and many people in similar circumstances. Group psychotherapy with people affected in like fashion seemed to be the most likely modality to fulfill these purposes.

THE IMPACT OF PSYCHOTHERAPY

By the time Mary had recovered significantly to the point where she could truly participate and use psychotherapy, our

Clozaril Feelings Group had been meeting for about two years. We were thrilled by the idea of including Mary in our psychotherapy group. We believed we were offering her the gold standard of treatment for those wishing to understand and experience themselves differently. Her reaction to our suggestion was unanticipated. She appeared offended, but agreed, grudgingly, to come to a session and see how that went. After one meeting at which she spoke very well and was well received by the other recovering patients, she refused to return, complaining that her feet hurt and it was too far to walk. When a staff member offered to pick her up and bring her by car, she professed to have a tenants' meeting at the same time that she could not miss. Mary finally admitted that she did not like groups because people in groups made her feel more insecure than people one at a time.

Many months later, after much work by her case manager, Mary finally agreed to make a commitment to group psychotherapy. During the meetings she spent as much time as possible talking about her painful feet, her bowel trouble, and her wish for more medication. It took a great deal of confrontation and repetition of requests to defer concerns about her body and medication to the medication group. Attempts during this interval to interpret to Mary and the group her possible reasons for focusing on somatic complaints and the menu of pills that she wanted met with denial and irritation, or alternately she felt hurt and misunderstood.

After many months that felt like running in place, Mary quipped one day, at last, "Well, I guess I'm going to have to talk about my feelings." And she indeed talked about her feelings. There were very few relapses back to somatic preoccupations. The presence in her group of her case manager was critical in helping her summon the courage and persistence to talk about her feelings. She talked about her disappointment in her son who was abusing drugs and belonged to a satanic cult and her agony over being unable to have been a better mother. She grieved her mother's growing infirmity and anticipated death. She mourned her own loss in not having had a normal life. After much work in her group, she began to really attend a tenants' meeting with a new friend, her attention to her appearance was remarkably better, and she began to travel and shop independently. She stopped asking for more pills and admitted that she had been feeling better since her medications were simplified to monotherapy with Clozaril alone.

WHAT TO DO WITH A LIFE FREE OF RATS

The rat lady of Bridgeport had achieved a great deal. She had been given a new lease on life by taking a wonder drug. Yet there is no doubt that her life would have remained confined to somatic preoccupations as she was fearful and avoidant of filling her life with enrichening experiences. Free of her rats, she was terribly lonely; her life was empty and disappointing, and she was without hope of replacing her career as a mental patient with an expanded identity and a new design for living. Psychotherapy was decisive in helping her enter a multidimensional recovery that brought her joy and satisfaction.

7

John's American Pie

A long, long time ago
I can still remember how that music used to make me smile
And I knew if I had my chance that
I could make those people dance and
maybe they'd be happy for a while.

So, bye-bye, Miss American Pie
Drove my Chevy to the levee but the levee was dry.
Them good ole boys were drinkin' whiskey and rye
Singin' this'll be the day that I die,
This'll be the day that I die.

Don McLean, American Pie

GETTING TO KNOW A SEVERELY MENTALLY ILL PERSON

Seeing people in community mental health centers ten or fifteen years into pervasive mental illness offers little opportunity to know what they were like before they developed schizophrenia or other severe treatment-resistant psychosis. The people affected by progressive mental illness rarely preserve the capability to reveal themselves as they were during childhood or adolescence. Their communication skills are eroded along with their cognition. Clinicians are reliant upon archived medical records or the accounts of family.

Past case records are inconsistently helpful in reaching an understanding of what a person was like before the illness became the foundation of the way he or she formed a sense of identity. Archived psychiatric medical records are sometimes unfindable, incomplete, or illegible. Family members are inconsistently reliable as informants for various reasons. When they are not totally burned out and unavailable for interview, they may not want to recover painful memories of what their son or daughter, sister or brother was like before mental illness robbed them of their original potential. Such memories are agonizing. Family members may also be hesitant to discuss a loved one's preillness life. Having a mentally ill person in the family is often regarded as embarrassing and shameful. Until mental illness is fully accepted on a par with physical illness, the associated stigma will carry the potential for a very distorted or irretrievable remembrance of what is lost and can never be found. Therefore, mental health clinicians face impediments in forming a complete view of who the patient was, is, and has the potential to become.

Sometimes, however, we are fortunate. Patients may have retained the ability to explain who they were and who they have become, or with treatment they recover vital cognitive function and with that a resumed capacity to tell us what they were like before the onset of mental illness. Archived psychiatric records may be found, complete or almost complete, legible, and written by a good clinician. Family members may be able to tell us more then they want to remember.

WHAT DIDN'T HAPPEN

Contrary to what many psychiatric professionals may think, people with schizophrenia often led pre-illness normal and ordinary lives. They were not crazy all their lives from day one. Nor do they have "poor protoplasm." Many do not come from crazy families. Their mothers did not pick them out from among their siblings and institute a major effort to drive them crazy. A few crazy families definitely do stand out. They draw lightning from clinicians, and conclusions about schizophrenogenic families are broadly overgeneralized. Theodore Lidz and colleagues (1965) and Alanen (1966) epitomize overgeneralized and frequently unempathic thinking about the families of people with schizophrenia, though they were not the only people who supported this type of thinking. Their thinking about families of schizophrenics has been replaced by that of others who observe the stressfulness of schizophrenia for victim and co-victims (families and close friends) and similarities between the reaction to schizophrenia and to other severe psychosomatic illnesses.

WHAT DID HAPPEN

The formation of goals and aspirations and the efforts to establish an identity during the teen years were aborted by the illness that gradually prevented people with severe schizophrenia from completing important developmental processes. Lidz and Lidz (1982) were correct in observing that "the patient had never adequately surmounted the critical developmental tasks of adolescence" (p. 8). The most dominant task of adolescence is that of establishing an identity. The focal questions an adolescent must answer according to the work of Kestenbaum (1993) are "Who am I," "What am I," and, "Where am I going?"

Lidz and Lidz (1982) describe the identity formation of mid- and late adolescence as a "lengthy process of separation from parents to achieve individuation as reasonably well-integrated, self-sufficient, and self-directed persons capable of relating intimately with someone outside the family" (p. 8).

Now and then we encounter patients in community mental health center practice who can still tell us who they are—that is, how far they got in forming a core sense of self—either by dint of having a less pervasive or less rapidly deteriorating form of schizophrenia or because they were not ill long enough (for less than ten years). Occasionally, we may also see patients whose positive symptoms (delusions and hallucinations), though entwined, may disclose something about their pre-illness interests and potential.

THE SIGNIFICANCE OF HALLUCINATIONS AND DELUSIONS

Hallucinations and delusions, though unanalyzable in the classical sense and by definition unamenable to reason, often contain clues or indicators about persons' central identity before illness overcame them. We are describing patients with lifelong, disabling schizophrenia who have negative and positive symptoms that persist. Also, there are cognitive impairments. The patients are not able to tell us about themselves in words free of hallucinations and delusions. A person who feels bugs and rats are devouring his brain and viscera is different from a person who believes he wrote a famous song.

The abolishment of expressive psychotherapy from community mental health centers is concordant with the decreased enthusiasm, and perhaps also insufficient training, to pursue an understanding of the patient through one or two key delusions. After ten years of illness, patients affected by severe schizophrenia have convoluted and interconnected delusions. Finding one or two central issues that would tell us something meaningful about the patient's core identity is frequently not an easy task.

Hallucinations are usually narrower in content than delusions. By inference, understanding the meaning of hallucinations should be easier. Yet hallucinations can be difficult to fathom because of their paucity of content.

We are not advocating that clinicians attempt to analyze hallucinations and delusions in the dynamic sense. Rather, we favor using the central delusions and to a certain extent key repetitive hallucinations as a guide to enabling each recovering patient to form an identity and lead a meaningful life.

NO "JOHN DOE"

John was no ordinary person. He was 22 years old when he was admitted to the Assertive Community Treatment Program for people with serious, treatment-resistant schizophrenia and noncompliance. By that time, he had been mentally ill without a complete remission from treatment for six years. John had been hospitalized twelve times with the frequency of hospitalization clearly increasing and with diminishing function. He had not worked in four years and was socially isolated, and his family had disconnected from him because he had assaulted his siblings, threatened his mother, and believed that she was putting things in his food and drink. At times he was certain that she was not his mother, but an impostor. He had been inducing himself to vomit because of his belief that he was being harmed by food and drink that she had prepared. In addition, he was pouring rubbing alcohol and stewed tomatoes into water glasses. John had been taking a baseball bat with him everywhere, including into the bathroom. His family was afraid of him, saw that his condition was worsening, and had lost hope that he could ever get any better.

Yet, even during a very intense exacerbation of his mental illness when he was severely psychotic, disorganized, and had porous ego boundaries, John conveyed his sense of being unique. He believed that he was a famous song writer and musician. In fact, he was convinced that he had written the

song "American Pie." Though he was unable to describe what
his beloved song was about, he was clear that the lyrics held
special significance to him, and he had loosely associated ideas
about having fathered a child with a girl named Heather who
then rejected him in favor of another man. The rejection by
Heather and the feeling that he had died appeared in fragmented and incomplete sentences. John did not know of
Heather or his child's whereabouts, yet he kept seeing her
unexpectedly throughout the streets of Bridgeport. He alternately believed himself to be a homosexual and said that his
father forced him to have anal intercourse with him and with
dogs. The homosexuality theme was not integrated with his
ideas about his relationship with Heather. His ideas about
homosexual-incestuous and bestiality experiences had a life of
their own. However, John did admit that he was confused
about whether the sexual experiences with his father and with
dogs really happened. He was confused about his relationship
with "Heather" and would only speak openly about his perceptions during worsening courses of his illness.

    John was positive at all times that he had written "Amer-
ican Pie." John maintained that the tune and lyrics had been
stolen from him. He brooded over not being given any money
or recognition for having written and sung this famous hit. He
could not remember the name of the man who was given
credit for authorship of "American Pie" or who sang the
popular hit. Similarly, he could not recollect any of the words.
The meaning of the lyrics was also not within his capacity to
describe. He became upset when asked specific questions
about "American Pie." "If you don't believe me, I'll find the
words I wrote. . . . There were other songs. . . . Maybe I can't.
. . . They were taken too." John had a theory that a car accident
had robbed him of his memory and that these strange experiences were caused by the resultant head injury. Alcohol abuse,
which had become a problem during his teen years, was a
continuing active issue. However, John did acknowledge a

problem with drinking, attended some Alcoholics Anonymous meetings, and was trying to become abstinent.

Obtaining a Socially Valued Role

Earlier in his illness, between hospitalizations, John had worked for brief periods of time at jobs as a mover and delivery man. Yet, it was also his desire to write popular songs with social significance or to resume his lost aptitude that led John to accept the case management and intensive rehabilitation program. His emphatic denial of mental illness or that he needed medication continued despite his cooperation with most treatment recommendations. Work planned for him at a social club run by people with mental illness proved to be an obstacle to his attainment of future goals, however. He refused to participate because the other clients were "sick" (mentally ill).

Unwilling to begin a vocational rehabilitation program in which he would follow the usual method of relearning the basics in a less stressful and structured environment that had an excellent track record at helping recovering patients obtain paid and sometimes competitive employment, John had a bleak vocational outlook. In an attempt to get him back in touch with performing music, he was introduced to another patient who really was writing and performing songs. While John did accept the introduction and agreed to meet the songwriter, who was also recovering from severe mental illness, to "jam," he wasn't able to strum even a simple chord on the guitar. Meanwhile, he insisted that he was a famous rock star who was playing his guitar with a famous band. He continued to express dismay that he was not receiving any pay yet. The vocational rehabilitation had reached an impasse.

However, John did achieve other important goals. He was able to live in an apartment with a roommate who was also recovering from severe mental illness, to control aggression toward his family, and to re-establish a connection with them although it was fragile and inconsistent. He was able to help his mother with her shopping and caring for his younger siblings. She had to be present all the time, however.

In addition, he continued to require help in performing activities of daily living. Financial support was provided by the state welfare system, and he required continuous supervision and guidance with money management. His apartment was always a mess, and he was unable to learn to cook beyond heating TV dinners. He was abusing alcohol at this time, seven or eight beers at least once a week; yet his alcohol use during this interval was substantially less than his former pattern. He enrolled in a course at a community college, but he suffered a setback, becoming disorganized, anxious, and delusionally preoccupied. He refused to complete the course or accept the help of a tutor. John had developed a severe movement disorder from his medication that was not relieved by standard treatments. Rapid involuntary movements affected his whole body. The hand and arm tremor may have made many activities of his daily life more difficult to complete and more frustrating. He was unable to make friends, though socialization with his family, roommate, and rehabilitation clinicians had improved. The preoccupation with being a rock star, having written "American Pie," and not being paid for his effort continued to have a life of its own, undaunted by medication.

In certain ways his condition worsened. He now believed that he had written many songs and albums, but was never recognized for his work. He blamed an upset stomach on a small rock he had eaten about a month ago. John explained, "I had to eat the rock to cleanse myself." His delusions were definitely expanding. He came to believe that a woman he had slept with recently dressed him up as a girl in the course of the night, and they made a musical video together in England. Preoccupation with royalties from the music intensified. He made frequent references to being shot in the mouth, with the bullet still imbedded in the back of his head.

Personal Despair

There seemed to be no way back for John. He aspired toward some ordinary goals such as loving and working. Yet he thought of himself as special, as a famous rock star who had written a moving and commercially successful tune. John wanted a socially valued role and considered himself distinctive from other people. He spurned the identity of a mental patient. There was no way he would believe what others told him. He hated his mother for treating him like he was crazy.

Yet, the song "American Pie" bore specific emotional meaning for him although he could not remember the content.

> I met a girl who sang the blues and
> I asked her for some happy news,
> But she just smiled and turned away,
> I went down to the sacred store
> where I heard the music years before
> But the man there said the music wouldn't play.
> And in the streets the children screamed,
> the lovers cried and the poets dreamed.
> But not a word was spoken
> the church bells all were broken.
> And the three men I admire most,
> the Father, Son and the Holy Ghost,
> They caught the last train for the coast the day the
>   music died.

Frustration everywhere. No replenishment from girls, music, children, poets, or from his religious life. Girls, music, the poetry of music and perhaps the poetry of life, and a spiritual life had been important to him.

During the interval of worsening psychosis, John's

American pie was unreachable. The girl turned away. The church bells were broken. The Holy Trinity left, never to return. The music died. He was without hope of acquiring any part of the American dream.

More about the American Dream

Don McLean spoke from the heart about what growing up in America was really like for many people. In the 1960s and 1970s Americans had an expectation of unlimited opportunity with the potential of having everything. The belief that all people can get their "American Pie," especially if they are willing to work hard and do what is expected, has persisted to a certain extent. Americans hook into the American ideal of getting something much larger than what they grew up having and in being able to reinvent the self. In contrast, Europeans, Asians, and people from Third World countries grow up knowing that expectations are limited by socioeconomic factors. These factors are usually outside the range of what they can control or change. In those countries, it is unlikely that a son or daughter can supersede a parent in career development or marital or monetary success. Usually they are obliged by financial and social constraints to enter the same business or occupation as their family. A certain amount of illness is anticipated. Relatives who are sick are cared for. For these reasons, it is not as crushing or diminishing to become ill in other countries. The sense of failure and profound personal despair that McLean describes in his powerful song is more likely to be felt by John and countless others who grew up believing that they would have their "American Pie."

Benefits of Clozapine

After almost ten years of progressive and increasingly pervasive mental illness, John accepted a trial of a newly available medication. The novel antipsychotic, Clozaril, had helped other people with persistent, increasing paranoid delusions and intense (though confined) feelings.

After several months of clozapine treatment, John began to look like a normal person. He stopped shaking. His rage was transformed into legitimate anger over being robbed of his youth and young adulthood. An ardent interest in his appearance resulted in his buying better clothes that showed a color consciousness. Serious plans to move to a new apartment in a better neighborhood in which there would be no exposure to alcohol and drugs from other tenants and neighbors were made and fulfilled. His social skills improved. He stopped drinking. The delusion about Heather dissolved. "Oh! That was just a weird idea. I don't think about that anymore." Violence was no longer in his realm of acceptable behaviors. No further hospitalizations were needed. John obtained a job in the competitive marketplace working as a courier for an investment firm. Good evaluations and promotions followed.

One year after initiating treatment, John admitted that he may not have written "American Pie": "I might have been confused." But he was still lonely and depressed, rejected the reality that he had a mental illness, and was filled with regrets that he had messed up his life and disappointed his family by drinking and smoking marijuana. He spoke openly about these feelings, but often commented that he had various insecurities and feelings that were difficult to talk about.

With the recovered capacity to reflect on his feelings rather than just experiencing them, it was now likely that John could benefit from expressive and perhaps exploratory psychotherapy.

Finding Words

John readily accepted group psychotherapy although he did not like groups and did not believe he had a mental illness. He participated fully and did not miss one session. Putting his feelings into words, finding out what he liked to do when he no longer had delusions to fill his time, and developing goals occupied him in a productive way. He spoke of his confusion about whether people were laughing at him and talking about him unkindly at work. He remembered that before he took Clozaril he used to be sure they were reading his mind and conspiring to harm him. He was able to engage in a discussion about the difference between cruel joking at another's expense and kidding a person as a way of telling that person you like him. The other group members expressed warm feelings toward him, which seemed to surprise and embarrass him. Yet he clearly listened to their feedback, conveyed appreciation, and seemed to benefit from hearing others share with him their perceptions of how they experienced him. The other group members admired him because he had gotten his life together, had his own apartment, and had obtained a job in the world of competitive employment.

After six months of group psychotherapy, he said he wanted to work on things by himself for a while. He indicated that his job had become very important to him. He had been asked to assume some supervisory responsibilities. The promotion was accompanied by a salary increase. It made him feel very satisfied. His relationships with co-workers had improved. He felt more secure around them and was able to deal with jokes at his expense without his thinking becoming disorganized and his mood caving in. At this time John spoke in complete sentences. He agreed that affectively charged thoughts and feelings, such as about dating and his music, could still derail his thinking. But his self-esteem suffered less, as he now understood this event better and knew that his thinking becoming temporarily disorganized did not mean that he was a bad person or that he was crazy.

Along with John's promotion, he agreed to work more hours. This meant that he could no longer come to the group. The other members expressed their sense of loss, but praised

John's achievements. One member remarked that since he saw John accomplish so much, he had gotten hope that his own life also could become more fulfilling. Another group member had developed a crush on John. Although she was unable to speak of her feelings in front of him, she missed him as well.

Some American Pie

Women, music, a car, a home of his own, appreciation, a job, and a sense of being an important person do not equal happiness. Yet John had accomplished a lot and was adjusting to a new sense of self. By this time he recognized that he had recovered suddenly and unexpectedly from severe mental illness.

He commented that as an adolescent, before the onset of mental illness, he had imagined that he would finish college and enter the criminal justice field like his father. However, he did not just want to be an ordinary police officer like his father. Rather, he dreamed of becoming a high-level administrator or professor in a law school. He also thought he would marry a beautiful girl, settle down in a house with a white picket fence, have a dog and two cars, and have friends with whom he would write and perform successful music. John expressed regrets about not achieving his ideal goal. He had hoped that taking a wonder drug would cure his schizophrenia. He had believed that a cure for his mental illness or entering a significant recovery would automatically bring him the whole "American Pie," that is, total fulfillment. John had to adjust not only to a sense of self changed by his illness and recovery experience that enabled a resumption of many faculties but he also had to perform the work of late adolescence and early adulthood. Setting reasonable and ego-compatible goals is not a smooth-functioning or painless process. Rather, it is often painful, confusing, and frustrating. John suffered. Yet he persisted in defining and adjusting to his sense of self as he emerged from severe mental illness during his late twenties through group psychotherapy. To a lesser but still significant extent during individual sessions he also worked on identifying feelings, defining what is normal experience, and reducing his expectations to fulfillable dreams.

8

The Mad Italian

Orestes never was Orestes, except in the periods when the Erinyes [furies or avenging gods] goaded him to insanity. Or the brief moments of respite from madness, as when he rested his head on a stone on a small island off Gythion. . . . Or in that suffocating place in Arcadia where he realized that he could no longer bear the Erinyes, or rather not so much them, for he had lost all hope of being rid of them, but their color, that impenetrable black in the noonday brilliance, and in exasperation he bit off a finger of his left hand. Upon which the Erinyes turned white.

But this reprieve didn't last long. Even when they were white they terrified him, more than before maybe, and they never stopped following him, despite falling asleep sometimes, despite taking wrong turns, slovenly but stubborn. He would see them plunging toward him, like bits of statues falling from the sky. And sometimes, as once along the gloomy bank of the Taurides, the terror was too much for him and he began to howl like a dog: a herd of white calves came toward him and Orestes thought they were all Erinyes, closing in around him.

Roberto Calasso, *The Marriage of Cadmus and Harmony*

Few descriptions of madness can surpass the spell-binding and macabre account of Orestes. His madness and persecution by the Furies followed one of the most violent and socially reprehensible crimes known to humanity. Orestes killed his mother, Clytemnestra and her lover Aegisthus, by the order of Apollo, as retribution for their murder of Orestes' father.

Although performed by the command of a god, and perhaps influenced by insanity, Orestes' actions were nevertheless condemned by the gods. Despite the guilt of the victims and the help given in committing this abhorrent act by his sister Electra and his friend Pylades, the avenging gods seized upon Orestes, persecuted him, and drove him frantically from land to land (Bulfinch 1942).

Nando, a man living in the 1980s in Bridgeport, Connecticut, who suffered from lifelong, disabling insanity, was also a tormented man. He felt that insects ate his brain and guts. Revolting though unseen animals hissed and howled at him day and night. Although Nando is not a man with the stature of the son of a commander-in-chief of an army or head of state, there are striking similarities to the plight of Orestes. Sex, violence, madness, homelessness, and intense persecution by persistent, horrifying nonhumans are all characteristics of Nando's and Orestes' condition. Neither Orestes nor Nando could find peace of mind, rest, or fulfillment in work or a loving relationship. Nando communicated his terror day and night. His frightening visions did not let him rest despite the major tranquilizer he was taking to relieve his suffering.

SEX, DRUGS, VIOLENCE, AND MENTAL ILLNESS

Clinicians no longer believe in the power of the gods to punish us by inflicting madness. We seek other explanations for insanity. Our explanations must include behaviors that seem to be causally linked with mental illness, though we may not always be certain which way the arrow of causality points. Do drugs and exposure to violence during early childhood and/or excessive or inappropriate sexuality cause mental illness, or does mental illness cause people to take drugs, become violent, and have poorly modulated sexual behavior? Clinicians are often confounded. We may learn the answer only after years of working with a mentally ill person, if at all. Because of the importance of sex, drugs, and violence in understanding and treating the severely mentally ill, and the barriers to providing psychotherapy to patients who are sexually inappropriate, high on drugs, and/or violent, we summarize in this chapter some of our observations and the findings from studies of people with mental illness who are violent, often abuse drugs, and have problems with the expression of their sexuality.

Drugs

Clinicians at staff meetings and conferences often bemoan the good old days when people with mental illness only had one diagnosis. Conference agendas and professional literature also attest to the widespread concern and the difficulty treating people who are dually diagnosed—substance abuse and schizophrenia or bipolar disorder.

In their paper about substance abuse among patients with treatment-resistant schizophrenia, Peter Buckley and colleagues (1994a) comment that 50 percent of patients with schizophrenia may have engaged in major abuse of alcohol or illicit drugs at some stage before or during the course of their illness. They also note, however, that reported estimates of the prevalence of such abuse vary substantially. In a related paper about substance abuse and clozapine treatment Buckley and colleagues (1994b) describe the impact of Clozaril on the 25 percent of their sample who also abused illegal drugs or alcohol. Substance abusers and nonabusers showed similar improvements on measures of psychopathology and psycho-social functioning after six months of clozapine therapy. Their conclusions are that clozapine may attenuate the craving for alcohol or cocaine in schizophrenic patients with co-morbid substance abuse. Our clinical experience confirms their find-ings.

However, the prevalence of co-morbid substance abuse in our patient population is nearer to 60 percent. Follow-up of our activity-oriented recovering patients shows that, despite the remission of substance abuse and the relief of schizo-phrenic symptoms, patients may feel rudderless and drift along without a sense of purpose or without much to occupy the empty spaces in their lives. Psychotherapy may help them find a sense of self, even if their self-definition lies in finding significant work and the skills to ensure their success. Since we do not have the means to determine who can be helped by psychotherapy and who cannot improve and meet desired goals with this modality, it is of vital importance to offer psychotherapy routinely to all people who are suddenly re-covering after years of persistent psychosis.

Violence

Much more has been written about the relationship between violence and mental illness than that between sexuality and mental illness. Kenneth Tardiff (1992) has noted the higher rates of violence among young male patients and patients in certain diagnostic groups. People with schizophrenia are dis-proportionately represented in groups of patients who are violent toward other people just before and/or during psychi-atric hospitalization. Violent mentally ill patients may believe that people are threatening, persecuting, or in some other way trying to harm them. Tardiff views violence as a reaction to perceived threats. A persecutory delusion is often present and persistent over time.

Among psychiatric patients homicide is more common than death by bronchitis, emphysema, and asthma combined (Eichelman 1987). Violent and aggressive behaviors are highly prevalent among psychiatric patients and often result in institutionalization or other severe disruptions of occupational, societal, familial, or other social functions (Yudofsky et al. 1986). As can be expected, aggression also limits progress toward significant rehabilitation. Tardiff (1992) notes that because aggressive patients are a heterogeneous group evaluation of aggression as a symptom is required. He cautions that consideration of current and prior medication use is indispensable.

Yudofsky and collegues (1986) define four types of aggression:

1. verbal aggression
2. physical aggression against self
3. physical aggression against objects
4. physical aggression against others

All types of aggression can be viewed as harmful and restricting of the person's broader self-definition or ability to delineate and accomplish future goals. Even verbal aggression, as opposed to assertiveness, can short-circuit significant communication. The extremes of verbal aggression such as yelling, menacing gestures while yelling, swearing, name calling, and threatening words make others defensive and curtail deeper interpersonal transactions.

Patrick Corrigan and colleagues (1993) review these procedures to assist patients with inconsistent or semi-consistent control of aggression against others: verbal de-escalation; behavioral interventions such as token economy, positive reinforcement of a patient's prosocial behaviors; aggression replacement—for example, differential reinforcement, assertiveness training, activity planning, decelerative techniques

such as social extinction and self-controlled time-out; phar-
macotherapy; and lastly, physical restraints. Few verbal techniques help people with patterns of habitual aggression against
others to establish consistent self-regulation.

Clinical experience with patients who have been violent,
who have spent significant time in restraints and quiet rooms,
and who eventually have an opportunity to take Clozaril
reveals a spectacular reduction in violence. With better control
over destructive and fear-inspiring impulses, patients have a
greater opportunity to learn to identify and express intense
affects through such formal modalities as case management,
rehabilitation, and psychotherapy and informally through relaxed interpersonal exchanges and experience.

Sex

Clinicians who work with the severely mentally ill often
become inured to the sexuality of patients. This process can
take the form of not noticing that the patient has a sex life, even
if it is only with him- or herself. Not noticing that the patient
has a sexuality beyond gender is usually possible only if the
patient does not demonstrate overarousal or inappropriate
sexuality by masturbating openly or approaching others for
sexual exchanges.

If the patient is demonstrative of sexuality, clinicians
usually do notice, but frequently pretend not to. The reasons
for clinicians not noticing are presumably embarrassment,
their feeling that the sexual arousal is not the worst of the
patient's problems, or their training has not prepared them to
help the patient with a sexual difficulty.

Another reason why clinicians may not comment or
intervene is because certain sexual behaviors, while excessive
and intrusive, are viewed as being gender concordant. Often
clinicians do not seem to notice or make explicit their observations of extreme sexual expressivity as long as it is viewed as

gender role concordant. Therefore, open displays of sexual feelings such as public masturbation and some aggressiveness in gratifying sexual desires are often better tolerated in males than in females. In contrast, clinicians often tolerate seductiveness in dress, gestures, or words better from females than males as long as it is subtly provocative rather than overtly aggressive. Accordingly, clinicians are not likely to clarify their observations, confront patients, or redirect potentially maladaptive sexual expressivity as long as it is perceived as gender appropriate.

Francine Cournos and colleagues (1993) document the frequency of sexual encounters between the severely mentally ill by administering questionnaires and tracking HIV positivity. Sexual encounters include not only vaginal and/or anal intercourse but also any sexual contact that involves the exchange of body fluids. They have found a high frequency of sexual expressivity involving exchange of body fluids among the severely mentally ill. Degen (1982) discusses the impact of unwanted side effects of major tranquilizers (conventional neuroleptics) on patients' sexual performance. People who need to take conventional neuroleptics to relieve their symptoms may become noncompliant to avoid these unwanted side effects of their medication.

Clinical observations of patients by those who provide treatment in community mental health centers or inpatient units include the following forms of sexual behavior: fondling one another, masturbation, intercourse (anal and vaginal), fellatio, tribadism, exhibitionism, pedophilia, sexual harassment, rape, and exchange of sexual favors for cigarettes, candy, chewing gum, or money.

Patients do not stop being people once they become mentally ill. Like other people, they have sex lives. Like many other people they have difficulty finding and navigating the complex path between repression and global exhibition of feelings. Because the symptoms of mental illness capture so much of their attention, often beginning during adolescence, the intricacies of working out satisfactory mechanisms for the appropriate expression of sexuality may never be negotiated. Sex role stereotypes have undergone enormous changes in the past twenty years. People who became and remained mentally ill through two decades of rapidly changing customs and values of sexual expression have serious needs for help in assimilating these changes and forming adaptive behaviors. Similarly, clinicians, who may themselves be middle-aged and therefore raised during very different times, often experience some non-contemporary views and responses to changes in sex role behavior. Clinicians may need to update their own understanding of sex and gender role behaviors in order to best help their patients sort things out and develop reasonable and ego-compatible sexual expressivity.

Patients who are affected by severe mental illness that is incompletely remitted often have difficulty expressing themselves in a way that is free enough of distortions to be understood by clinicians. Alternately, they may be too cognitively disorganized to communicate their feelings clearly, or they may hear clinicians' responses to them in distorted ways. With adequate symptom relief from newer medication, people unable to modulate the expression of their sexuality and previously also unable to talk about sex (a frequent dyad) retrieve the capacity to use language for self-expression and meaningful dialogue with others. Clinicians must not miss this valuable opportunity for significant psychotherapeutic intervention, even though the patient may no longer be attempting to rape people or sexually molest children. Clozaril helps people like Nando control such inappropriate sexual behavior as masturbating publicly and sexually harassing the clinicians. However, while poorly regulated exhibitionistic sexual behavior no longer occurred, Nando then retreated into his room with girlie magazines and spent the day alone smoking cigarettes, listening to music, and masturbating in private. This was undoubtly an improvement, but a far cry from satisfactory sexual expressivity. Expressive therapy was needed to help him reshape the fulfillment of sexual desire.

Sexual Orientation

Most people need to express themselves sexually, even if the expression is confined to self-soothing through sexual fantasy and masturbation. In our society people are generally assumed to be heterosexual whether they have a partner or are unpartnered unless proven otherwise. Proof of homosexuality may consist of self-disclosure (coming out), being disclosed by others (being outed), or observed homosexual activity.

The same norms for deciding who is straight and who is gay are followed for the mentally ill. However, suffering from low esteem, and low social value and struggling for some form of acceptance, it is not surprising that the mentally ill often disavow homosexuality, either as a core sexual identity or as a situational sexual feeling—one that is not a first-choice activity or a part of their self-definition. Accomplishing self-acceptance as a gay, lesbian, or bisexual is especially complex and troublesome for a person who has progressive and disabling schizophrenia that began in adolescence.

The prevalence of homosexuality among the lifelong mentally ill is not known. Situational homosexual behavior seems to be widespread, especially in such institutional settings as state hospitals or jails. Institutions routinely limit access to existing heterosexual partners, potential partners, and sexually explicit magazines or videos. Frequent opportunities for sexual expression with a partner are often limited to same-sex encounters. While our culture continues to accord the highest social value to heterosexuality and to stigmatize homosexuality overtly or covertly, people challenged by severe mental illness will have extra difficulty sorting out and expressing their sexual orientation and preference.

Clinicians often feel that sexual presentation needs to be muted or buffered and only react when sexuality is welded to aggression or seductive behavior or attire. The sexually aggressive are stereotypically male, whereas the seductive are stereotypically female. However, the less one abides by stereotypes in observing and understanding people, the more exceptions to the rule become apparent. We have certainly seen many females who harass or molest men, other women, or children, as well as men who are seductive in attire (wearing very tight pants, especially in the groin area, and showing bare legs, arms, and chest as if they were visiting the gym or beach), in gestures, or in words. Clinicians often seek to have those patients control their impulses and settle for containing sexual demonstrativeness without imparting a sufficient understanding or redirection of healthy impulses and drives.

Those who are sexually controlled or repressed often have no attention paid to their legitimate needs for sexual expression. Psychotherapy can be a very useful adjunct to case management and treatment with novel antipsychotics, especially as the psychosis resolves and new feelings can be clarified and understood.

Beyond Violence, Drugs, and Sex

Inappropriate sexual expressivity, drugs, and violence, in combination or alone, are problematic for mentally ill people and those who provide care to them. Providing psychotherapy for a patient whose self-control has diminished below acceptable boundaries is impossible, though we know the value of verbal de-escalation techniques. Verbal approaches to reducing threatening behavior are worthwhile, but cannot create a candidate for insight-oriented psychotherapy while a patient continues to have intense psychotic symptoms that are unrelieved by conventional treatment. We feel that more effective medication such as Clozaril is needed to diminish delusions, hallucinations, or such side effects as akathisia. When the patient is more comfortable and when staff are no longer apprehensive about being assaulted, psychotherapy can then be offered with the reasonable expectation of success. Violent, sexually preoccupied, and "druggie" mentally ill patients can also make use of psychotherapy, even if the outcome is to redirect their activity toward finding a self-definition in a job or hobby.

And, yes, this long preamble has a great deal to do with "the mad Italian."

BACK TO NANDO

Nando was raised in Stratford, Connecticut, in a middle-income family. His father was an immigrant from Italy who worked as a tailor until he retired. Nando's mother held steady employment as a factory worker. He had not seen his mother in five years at the time of admission to the Assertive Community Treatment Program. His father remained interested in him, but saw him infrequently. He was the fifth of six children.

His four sisters and one brother did not maintain contact with him. The reason for their discontinuing a relationship with Nando was unclear from his explanation or from his medical record. Among reasonable or educated guesses are that he had been verbally and physically assaultive to them, influenced by his double problem of drug abuse and worsening schizophrenia. There is a sentence in his record about his violence toward his family. "He hit his mother in the jaw" while vague, irrational, delusional, and hallucinating. During this time, he was abusing LSD, mescaline, speed, marijuana, and alcohol.

Nando's problem with drugs began at age 16. There is no evidence of impairments in achieving developmental milestones and he completed eleventh grade. After leaving school, Nando worked at factory jobs, often being laid off after several months of work. Although he got other jobs, the capacity to obtain and maintain employment diminished after the appearance of schizophrenia and continued drug abuse.

During the managed deinstitutionalization of Connecticut state hospitals, after multiple psychiatric hospitalizations of increasing length, including a seven-year stay after an assault on his mother, Nando was admitted to an assertive community treatment program. By then he was 40 years old. After admission to this program, he continued to hallucinate, be delusional, and have continuous paranoid thoughts of insects eating him. He often participated in same-sex encounters for a few cigarettes or fifty cents. Nando was easily exploited financially as well as sexually. He would often sell a television or expensive stereo for a pack of cigarettes. His lack of self-control culminated in an attack upon his case manager because of delusional and hallucinatory behavior that did not resolve with standard antipsychotic treatment. He believed that he was being driven out of his apartment. The clinician he struck is a gentle man, capable, direct, and trustworthy, who is loved and revered by other patients. Nando also assailed other patients.

He often asked to return to the state hospital when he felt lonely, disconnected, out of control, and frightened of the higher demands made of him by living in an apartment rather than a state hospital. Nando also frequently told staff that his sex life was better at the state hospital. There he was able to have as much sex as he wanted with a partner, though usually a same-sex partner. He seemed to find these encounters less intimidating than heterosexual sex, though he did not identify himself as homosexual and preferred "girlie" magazines for masturbatory satisfaction. Nando's sexual preoccupation increased. He often masturbated constantly and in public places and became verbally abusive whenever staff members attempted to discuss the subject with him. During the time of

worsening schizophrenia, an old problem that had become
dormant resurfaced: Nando began to drink water obsessively.
His blood sodium level plummeted, putting him at continuous
risk of seizures and possibly increasing his irritability. He was
frequently verbally and physically abusive to staff, sexually
harassed female staff, and during an effort to bring him peace-
fully to an area of the outpatient department that would be less
stimulating, he threw two staff members who were trained in
martial arts across the lobby. Nando got his wish to return to
the state hospital after decompensating further and after assaulting his kind and sensitive case manager.

PSYCHOSIS AND RACISM

Although not the core of our chapter about Nando's madness,
racism is linked with Nando's life as a mentally ill person who
experienced worsening schizophrenia. Nando was not overtly
racist during stable intervals. However, the duration of his
stable periods was growing shorter and the precipitant of
increasing psychosis less apparent. Nando was a person who
spoke and acted like a racist when his impulses were blazing
and ego structures were porous and inconsistent. Calasso's
(1993) eloquent account of Orestes' madness and persecution
by the Furies speaks of that mad man's racism: "he realized
that he could no longer bear the Erinyes, or rather not so much
them, for he had lost all hope of being rid of them, but their
color, that impenetrable black in the noonday brilliance" (pp.
190–191). Out of exasperation Orestes gnaws off a finger of
his left hand, and the Erinyes turn white. Orestes thereby
obtains his desired color transformation and a brief respite
from suffering. The subtext might read as follows: black
Erinyes are bad, and white Erinyes are good. Therefore, erad-
icate black people or transform them into white and you will
erase your suffering. In real life, however, racist beliefs are
generally unconfirmed just as they are in Calasso's stunning

account. The white Erinyes are no better: "even when they were white they terrified him, more than before maybe."

Orestes' racism was reincarnated during Nando's decompensations into intensified psychosis. However, he did not have to bite off his finger. To lessen his suffering, his black and women case managers were replaced by white males, and his torment increased, culminating in an assault upon a white male clinician.

Clinicians often observe a focus on and belittling of ethnic diversity by the mentally ill. This contempt often worsens as the patient becomes more disorganized. Thought content may be organized along a paranoid axis. In the case of a paranoid focus the disorganized patient may speak of "niggers" trying to rape or kill him. The black or African-American may speak of the "crackers" just trying to get his or her money or being sexually exploitive.

In *The Nature of Prejudice* Gordon W. Allport (1982) writes at length about prejudice and its many dimensions. He notes that those who hate themselves, especially when the hatred has been instilled in their unconscious by presumably multiple early life experiences, have the potential to uphold racist attitudes, even though they are inconsistent with reality.

The mentally ill are particularly prone to racist attitudes, as their self-loathing, developed through internalized societal values, is often profound. Nando is a person who while decompensating would say the most insulting things to black staff and other patients. He would order them around in a rude tone of voice as if they were subordinates, calling them "boy" or "whore." He was not able to listen to confrontation about his attitudes and comments to black staff, no matter how gentle. Similarly, he was not educable as he did not acknowledge any limitations to his understanding of racial differences and his thinking was very disorganized.

Allport's comments about the purpose of stereotyping others by some arbitrary characteristics are helpful in understanding Nando's needs. He views the stereotype as a selective device to maintain simplicity in perception and in thinking. While Nando was drifting further from reality and deeper into his delusional world of ghastly insects and animals eating his brains and guts, his thinking becoming progressively less coherent and his actions less organized, he desperately needed to latch onto some ideas about people that were simple, convenient (most of his clinicians were black or women), rigid, and deeply etched in his mind. Like many racists and sexists, he also had a bias against Jews and gay people.

You are probably wondering whether Clozaril can cure or lessen racism (and other nonconstructive "isms").

Is Clozaril a Racism Blocker?

Clozapine has many novel properties at the level of the brain chemoreceptor, and we do not know whether the new chemical profile of Clozaril offers hope of overcoming racism. Probably it would not be useful with garden-variety neurotic bigotry. However, it is striking in Nando and with other patients recovering suddenly from lifelong relentless mental illness that deeply entrenched and easily fixated-on derisive beliefs about ethnic differences do modify in intensity if not in substance. In tandem with the deflection of all-consuming prejudice by reducing aggressivity in general and by restoring other cognitive abilities, Clozaril does effectively optimize a recovering person's accessibility for the discussions, education, and healing of psychotherapy. All of these modalities can alleviate racism.

OUTCOME OF NANDO'S INVOLVEMENT IN ASSERTIVE CASE MANAGEMENT

Although Nando was offered the standard smorgasbord of programs and services as part of the wave of managed deinstitutionalization, his symptoms were not sufficiently diminished. His conventional medication was modified, and adjuvant medications were added, but no sufficient relief of symptoms occurred. His violence, alcohol abuse, intrusive sexual expressivity, racism, and low ability to learn self-promoted activities of daily living impeded his progress. Nando was destined to spend most of the remainder of his life in less natural environments such as acute inpatient care or state hospitals.

THE ROLE OF CLOZARIL IN NANDO'S LIFE

Although the insects devouring his brain and body cavities were very real to him, Nando was willing to expose himself to the risk of developing agranulocytosis and a weekly blood cell count to obtain Clozaril. He was dubious about the ability of medication to erase his torment. Nonetheless, he accepted a trial of clozapine, hoping that his suffering could be lessened and that he would be again able to get and hold a job. Both goals were as important to him as obtaining coffee, sex, and cigarettes.

After three months of Clozaril treatment Nando was able to contain aggressive feelings. His agitation was focused, and he was easily consoled or talked down. His desire to control excessive aggression and revise sexual expressivity was evident in his group psychotherapy. He commented one day while other group members were discussing dating and their like or dislike of sex that his case manager had objected to his "girlie" magazines because they made him masturbate "too much." Too much was most of the day, although this was a positive change because his self-soothing was limited to his bedroom, rather then the pre-Clozaril "anywhere and constantly." He heard the gentle confrontation with mingled sadness, irritation, and relief. The moderate limit setting must have offered him some valuable guidelines to living a normal life because he was able to understand the confrontation, modify his behavior to less frequent and "private time," and express his thoughts and feelings without evidence of obstructions to other group members. The group members listened, indicating their interest by looking at him during his disclosure and nodding empathically.

After six months, Nando's appearance had improved remarkably. He dressed in clean and very well-coordinated clothes that were fashionable. His personal cleanliness (no smell, hair and beard clean) and fashion-conscious clothing were apparent and appreciated. The little fan that had to be activated to blow unwanted odors the other way whenever Nando was in an enclosed space, such as a clinician's office entered the archives of Nando's history. His negative schizophrenic symptoms were finally, after many years of intensive effort, departing.

In accordance with these changes, Nando very often expressed how much he would like to work. He liked money, had pride in himself as fulfilling a socially valued role, and clearly enjoyed the praise the staff gave him for achieving his ambitions. After eight months of treatment with Clozaril and six months of group psychotherapy, although still afflicted by loose associations that made some of his speech difficult to follow, he got a job in the maintenance department of the agency.

There were some setbacks. Whenever his check came (once a month) or his case manager was away (during scheduled time off such as a vacation or conference), he became disorganized and intrusive and seemed to be decompensating, despite continuing an apparently minimum effective amount of Clozapine. The usual crisis-style interventions were offered successfully. Nando has never been rehospitalized or asked to be rehospitalized since initiating treatment with clozapine. His general behavior and ability to contain intense affective states have improved, and his ability to propose his feelings to his group and to clinicians has strengthened.

Nando asked to leave the group since he wanted to increase his hours at work. His job performance improved. He felt a sense of dignity in increasing his hours. His increased income gave him pleasure, extended self-interest, approval, and value. He was transferred to a bimonthly Clozaril support and medication monitoring and education group for people who were satisfied with the progress of their recovery, were stable, and were not interested in further self-reflection.

PSYCHOTHERAPEUTIC HEALING BY WORKING IN THE "PROXIMATE DEVELOPMENTAL ZONE"

Daniel Stern's (1985) work on understanding the thinking and behavior of parents and children and how to use that understanding to help them in therapy is not at all about people who have been severely mentally ill, violent, drugging, sexually preoccupied, or racist. Though Stern's findings seem to be very distant from our patients' struggles and our striving to help them, much of the information he has gleaned and made available to clinicians in his writing and lecturing is useful in our work.

In order to help people recovering suddenly from life-long mental illness, particularly those who define themselves by activity rather than by reflecting on their values and characteristics, Stern's notion of working with the patient in their *proximate developmental zone* has been critical to eliciting an enthusiastic response to psychotherapeutic engagement. Many of our action-prone patients had been offered traditional-style psychotherapy before and during recovery. By traditional-style psychotherapy we mean an emphasis on understanding transference, support of healthy ego components, bolstering self-esteem, and exploration of feelings by asking such questions as "How do you feel?" or making broad statements such as "You must have been very angry!" In general we find these therapeutic interventions to impede the patient's expressivity, causing them to clam up rather than open up.

The patients rejected these early attempts at therapy by not attending or leaving sessions early, presumably because they felt disconnected and unengaged. Working therapeutically very near where the patients' most urgent feelings lie is not easy, but is worth the effort. Asking action-directed patients who are admiring a painting on the wall what the picture means to them may be experienced as disconnecting and perhaps disintegrating or confusing because they do not know and do not have the verbal skill or motivation to reflect on their feelings in order to find out. It is much better for a therapist to comment to an activity-geared person that there are many ways to express feelings that are not verbal and painting is one of them. This comment led to a vivid discussion among group members about how they liked to express themselves in word-free activities before becoming mentally ill, and to muse over how they had lost significant activities throughout their years of mental illness. There was a suggestion from the group that the recapture or development of important self-defining activities might be a vital component of their strengthening sense of self and of obtaining pleasure from this world.

Indeed, Nando began to talk more and more about his desire to work. He invested more time in taking care of his roommate by preparing meals and keeping their apartment clean, and he took pride in his accomplishments. When he finally got a job working at the agency in the maintenance department, he announced that the voices that he heard coming from the vacuum were becoming fainter and less frequent. His concentration improved. He was asked to increase his hours and eventually graduated to less supervised employment for higher functioning people at the Kennedy Center, a job preparation and placement agency in Bridgeport. Instead of spending all his extra money on cigarettes and "girlie" magazines, he began to buy nice clothes. He took pleasure in his new look and in the many compliments he received.

Nando has made a major transformation. For years he had announced to the world his chaotic and agonizing mental life through violence, drinking, sexual preoccupation, and racist comments. He now is able to inform the world of his improved sense of self-worth and his more relaxed mental life by dressing well, working well, and respecting himself and others.

9

From Wild Men to Lambs

At the hole where he went in
Red-Eye called to Wrinkle-Skin.
Hear what little Red-Eye saith:
"Nag, come up and dance with death!"

Eye to eye and head to head,
This shall end when one is dead;
Turn for turn and twist for twist—
Hah! The hooded Death has missed!

Rudyard Kipling, *The Jungle Book*

In this chapter we continue to describe Clozaril's effect on various kinds of impulsivity. Easily and highly arousable people who are prone to unplanned, extreme, and frequently unpredictable actions seem to acquire the capacity for self-restraint during treatment with Clozaril. At this point they may benefit from psychotherapy and psychotherapy can be an important experience. It may help the patients identify a changing sense of self and to share this awareness openly.

From our experience patients seem to require an opportunity to express themselves in words in a place and situation where they are openly and formally acknowledged. Psychotherapy does not diminish their need for action. Rather, psychotherapy seems to help them utilize action, their usual modus operandi, at a higher level of organization to adjust to a changed sense of self.

THE WILD MEN

In this chapter we describe three patients with a tradition of violence, inappropriate sexual expressivity, and drug use. They are recovering from persistent and severe mental illness and have accepted psychotherapeutic intervention during their struggle to achieve a new sense of self with a socially valued role. Before taking Clozaril, these three "wild men" were fearsome, unpredictable, dangerous, and unproductive and were spending most of their time in acute care hospitals or the forensic units of the state hospital. On Clozaril alone, before group psychotherapy was added, they had become less aggressive and easier to console and were able to live outside the hospital for long periods of time. However, they required highly supervised housing and guidance with money and time management and nutrition. They spent most of their time smoking cigarettes alone in their rooms or walking aimlessly throughout the city of Bridgeport. They did not work. They did not speak to one another during their medication groups and spoke only to staff to ask for things they needed or in response to a question. They had no friends.

In the story "Rikki-tikki-tavi," Kipling (1894) uses strong language to convey the struggle between the mongoose "Red-Eye" (Rikki-tikki-tavi) and the cobra "Wrinkle-Skin" (Nag). Good and evil, right and wrong, triumph and death are so polarized that they are crystal clear and viscerally felt. We have no doubt who is evil and who is good in Kipling's evocative tale. We know who should triumph and who should die as soon as Kipling tells us about the cobra Nag, who ate the helpless fledgling that accidentally fell out of the nest. Nag then diverted Rikki's attention while his companion cobra, Nagiera, attempted to slither undetected toward Rikki from another direction to kill him without a fair fight. We know that Nag and Nagiera are wrong, and we are not surprised that the cobra, the hooded Death, struck and missed and would undoubtedly meet her own death instead.

Delusions often imitate Kipling's account of Nag, Nagiera and Rikki-tikki-tavi. Good and evil are clear. The people who are assaulted or killed well deserve it. In human, "real" life, however, good and evil are usually not clear. People who are assaulted or killed often do not deserve it. The mentally ill with paranoid delusions or command hallucinations can attack, harm, or kill another based on erroneous or distorted beliefs. The innocent who are harmed may never recover. The dead will never get back their life.

The jungle law is to kill only what you need for food or in self-defense. In the jungle and in most of the natural world, the jungle law is usually obeyed. Humans, however, who on some level experience similar polarized and viscerally felt occurrences as our not-so-distant relatives in the jungle, frequently kill or attempt to kill other humans for reasons other than food. We often kill out of greed, envy, or revenge. Also, we may kill or attempt to harm others because of distortions in our perception. That is, we may feel other people are trying to harm or kill us by dint of paranoid delusions or thoughts and feelings that are overdetermined. Such beliefs, though false— that is, either based upon overvalued ideas such as racism or on delusions—can, if acted on, cause harm to others through harassment or violence.

The people we are writing about in this chapter were wild men who injured other people because they felt unjustly threatened or persecuted. Though we understand their beliefs to be delusional, their perception of themselves and others were very plausible to them. The experience of Henry, Lance, and Ira before and after taking Clozaril is an intriguing story of wild men who became lambs. Yet, increasing their function from simply being mild-mannered and gentle to securing a position of value to family and others occurred only after the additional endeavor of psychotherapy.

ONE WILD MAN'S RAGE

While always difficult for his parents to handle, Henry came from an average middle-class African-American family. His mother, father, brothers, and sisters had achieved professional degrees and worked in managerial positions. There were good relationships among family members with the exception of Henry. He was always a "nervous" child. Until he reached the third grade he had received average school grades. Around this time he became very rebellious. He had the typical signs of a "black sheep." By the time he finished ninth grade he had become so difficult to handle that even a special education class did not foster satisfactory self-control or learning. His family had become burnt out, tired of his inability to control his anger. Verbal abuse and threatening gestures expanded to drinking, smoking marijuana, and inappropriate sexual expressivity. By age 17 he was smoking marijuana regularly and drinking a case of beer a day. He held jobs as a pipe cutter for a few weeks at a time, which usually culminated in being fired for arguing with his boss or being unwilling to follow instructions. Dating girls deteriorated into making unwanted and continuous sexual overtures to people in his community. He was placed in foster care or boarding homes as a ward of the state. All of his many placements ended in his being thrown out. His rage, obscene remarks, display of obscene literature, and chasing neighborhood girls made him unwelcome everywhere, and eventually he was rehospitalized. The six-year hospitalization prior to his admission to the managed deinstitutionalization program followed more than thirteen psychiatric admissions in ten years.

Although Henry had begun his career as a mental patient at age 16 in a private hospital, he quickly lost his private health insurance and his family's empathic support. They were often the target of his rage and rarely the focus of his appreciation. When asked about his presenting problem during admission to the community treatment program, in a rare effort to answer a question coherently, he said, "The pills. Just the pills. I don't want to talk to no damned doctor." His delusional thinking, hallucinatory behavior, agitation, verbal abuse of staff and other patients, threatening gestures, and inconsistent cooperation with his treatment did not bode well for his future. He could not tolerate group therapy or individual visits lasting more than a few minutes. He spent his days of less restrictive treatment—that is, out of the hospital—watching television, reading, and walking around the neighborhood, friendless and jobless. In a particularly tumultuous event just before he accepted a trial of Clozaril, Henry went berserk and trashed his room, smearing excrement and blood all over the mirrors and walls.

From Rage to Tranquility

Henry made extraordinary progress during his treatment with Clozaril. He became cooperative with staff in meeting his treatment goals. Formerly, his money management guidance would result in threats toward the staff who were helping him meet such desired goals as paying his rent. He wanted his entire check for his own immediate use, believing that staff or someone had stolen his "other" money that was intended for the rent. While taking his new medicine, he became cooperative with treatment, partially because he was no longer delusional and partly because his cognitive organization improved. He could recognize that his entitlement check included his rent. Henry's irritability lessened. He got himself a job stocking shelves and sweeping the floor at the corner grocery story near his apartment. His mother resumed a relationship with him and eventually invited him to Sunday dinner and other family activities. His brother and sister began to spend time with him after many years of estrangement.

Although Henry was doing better, he was not working many hours and still had a great deal of unstructured time. He would not participate in any activities at the mental health center. He had no friends.

Henry was one of the first ten patients to be offered Clozaril. He came to his medication group faithfully, although he would only sit for about ten minutes. He then asked if he could just get his medicine and leave. Staff found Henry to have some likable qualities, such as his desire to work and keep his apartment spotless, and he had a certain personal warmth. For these reasons it made sense to offer him group psychotherapy, although he was not high functioning in many ways and it was not clear whether Henry could progress further given his dislike of being with other people and his general unwillingness to converse with anyone.

A paradox in Henry's behavior did not escape us. While professing to dislike being with people and acting irritable whenever approached for any reason, when he had recovered sufficiently he got himself a job in a grocery store in which a considerable number of people came and went. Some of the customers must have tried to talk to him, even if only to ask him for things. Henry could have gotten a job at Goodwill where he would have been alone almost all the time. At first the staff were skeptical. They thought he must have been drawn to work in that store because of the easier access to drugs and alcohol that it afforded. Staff saw Henry every day at the store or in his apartment to monitor his self-administration of Clozaril. There was never any evidence that their concerns about drugs or alcohol had any grounds.

Did group psychotherapy help Henry? We will never really know the answer. When changes were made in the format of the medication group to transform it into one in which psychotherapy could be offered, Henry continued to participate. He came for about six months faithfully and willingly. He no longer asked to leave early. He answered questions with a few more words than "yes" or "no" and no longer sounded or appeared irritated. While Henry never developed the gift of gab or love of conversation, he did begin to talk sociably to the other patients in the group and to listen to them. He developed some "corner store friends" with whom he enjoyed being. He began to spend more time there, enjoying his work as well. His grooming improved. His mother, sister, and brother were spending more time with him and bought him nice clothing. He looked very elegant and took pride in his new look. Although he did not resume dating, he also did not have inappropriate sexual encounters. His interest in pornography remained a private matter.

To our surprise, Henry agreed to participate in our endeavor to make an educational video with Sandoz Pharmaceuticals about people who were recovering from serious, persistent mental illness. He listened while the consent form was read to him, signed without hesitation, and participated in the group session that was being taped, unruffled by the cameramen, lights, and audiotechnicians.

After six months of group psychotherapy, Henry said that he preferred to be transferred to a medication only program as he wanted to spend more time working in the corner store. Staff applauded his progress and agreed with his decision.

ATTILA THE HUN

Lance, a massively built young man, was 22 years old when he entered the Forensic Institute for the first time. He was charged with first-degree sexual assault. His psychiatric history began eight years before the sexual assault. By age 33 he had fifteen psychiatric hospitalizations for treatment of bizarre behavior, assaults, and the inability to care for himself due to disorganization, hallucinatory behavior, and delusions. When Lance was discharged into the intensive care community psychiatry program after many years of psychiatric hospitalization, he was considered very dangerous. It was uncertain whether he would be able to receive his treatment consistently enough under less restrictive circumstances of community outreach and support services.

Lance's admission to the community treatment program was controversial because of his dangerousness when decompensated, his instability, and his incomplete response to conventional neuroleptics including depot (injectable, long-acting) haloperidol. Lance's first three years in the community treatment program were checkered. Very low-functioning behavior, instability, unpredictable verbal abusiveness, menacing gestures, and refusal to take medicine were mingled with improvements in functioning and fewer episodes of verbal abuse or threats toward other people. He was able to get a job in the maintenance department of the facility where he was receiving treatment. He worked two to three days a week for several hours each day.

From Hell to Purgatory

However, Lance was in limbo. His journey from hell to purgatory was worthwhile, but hardly finished. He could not complete a grammatically correct sentence with subject, verb, and object. His pervasive thought disorder generated speech that was difficult to understand. His huge size and grotesque communication evoked disagreeable feelings. Lance was almost always shunned by other people.

From Purgatory to Group Psychotherapy

Early in his treatment with clozapine when his aggression was under improved self-containment, his level of organization had increased, and Lance was able to sit for a half-hour without being disruptive, he joined the psychotherapy group for people recovering from severe schizophrenia. During one session, he spoke of his attempt to date another member of his psychotherapy group. He had no prior history of dating nor any practice or obvious paradigm for the dating situation. Twenty years had passed since he was a teenager. The customs of dating had changed, and there was no evidence that he had ever even learned the outdated customs of dating well enough to apply them successfully. Nevertheless, Lance was clearly in the early stage of recovering from severe persistent mental illness, and he was able to ask a woman on a date. From his description we knew that he clearly recognized two aspects of dating. The first improvement in his cognitive function and impulse control was his recognition that when you feel attracted to someone you do not grab her at the first opportunity, throw her down, and force yourself upon her. Instead, you ask the person on a date. The second improvement was his ability to plan for the future. He knew where to go on a date (he asked her to have lunch at a local diner) and sent a clear socially appropriate signal that his invitation was a date, not simply having lunch with a friend. He accomplished this signaling by offering to pay for her lunch. The object of his interest had recovered remarkably after many months of treatment with clozapine and was further along in her recovery. However, she was still uncertain about relationships with men, among other things. She told the group that she resented the assumptions men make (not just Lance) while having lunch with a woman, particularly when they offer to pay for lunch and the offer is accepted. She mentioned that Lance had asked her to have lunch. She commented that accepting the free lunch did not mean that she was interested in doing "other things." Lance was a "touchy-feely" African-American. He probably had also tried to touch her beyond her liking. Yet there was no evidence of coercion or aggression. Lance had progressed many notches over his former "take what you want" impulsivity. Her rudimentary understanding of the customs surrounding dating, and his lack of sophistication in understanding her naiveté and ambivalence both resembled the early adolescent difficulty in sorting out the customs and structure of dating and gender-related differences.

We tried to explore their feelings, hoping that an enlarged understanding would lead to increased interpersonal skills. Both seemed soothed, but neither was interested in extending the exploration beyond one occasion or deepening a relationship with each other. Yet each of these action-accustomed people had participated in the group psychotherapy session with attention, expression of aggressive feelings in words, and containment of discourteous comments to each other. Lance was able to rise above his disappointment with the woman and focus his attention on his work. He increased his hours at work, and the quality of his performance improved. With only a few setbacks, Lance was able to get a job in a more prestigious sheltered work setting at the Kennedy Center. He accepted a position in the maintenance department that paid higher wages and was reserved for higher-functioning people. Lance has made extraordinary advances in his goal of finding significant work.

Staff and other patients have found Lance approachable and have been willing to spend more productive time with him. Rather than talking him down or putting him in restraints, staff are able to talk with him about how to get an apartment of his own, keep it clean, take better care of his own appearance, and do such "fun things" as fishing. Lance did indeed get his own apartment. This was the fulfillment of an important goal.

While group psychotherapy did not cure him, sorting and prioritizing his issues did occur. Lance felt pride in his success.

IRA THE TERRIBLE

Ira is a 40-year-old unemployed, never married, Hispanic man with a history of more than ten admissions to acute care psychiatric hospitals. His eleventh hospital admission prior to involvement in the community psychiatry program lasted nine years. Much of his inpatient stay took place at a forensic institute for the criminally insane. He had an extensive history of marijuana and alcohol abuse, exhibitionism, pedophilia, and assault. His problems were exacerbated during late adolescence when he developed schizophrenia. Ira was physically abusive toward his mother many times, usually when she tried to place limits on his behavior. His family had a high tolerance for his violence and drug abuse.

Ira's Life before Schizophrenia

Born in Puerto Rico, Ira had a life described by family as normal. He was one of six children. He achieved developmental milestones within normal limits. He did not do well in school, but was promoted within the usual timetable. Ira did not attend any special classes. He completed two years of high school. By this time he was drinking alcohol, smoking marijuana, and sniffing glue every day whenever possible. By age 18 he had dated girls and experienced sexual intercourse, but he did not have a steady girlfriend. Ira's history up to this point was unremarkable and did not differ from many inner-city young Puerto Rican men. Things began to change after his eighteenth birthday. His ability to get a date seemed to diminish, presumably because he had begun to make lewd comments and had become coercive. He became disorganized and his thinking and speech bizarre. His assaultiveness toward his family, particularly his mother, increased. He was only able to hold factory jobs for several months at a time. Since his second hospitalization he has not been able to work.

Last and Longest Hospital Admission

Ira's last and longest admission to the hospital was precipitated by exposing himself to a little girl. His violence continued throughout his hospitalization. He assaulted staff and other patients at the state hospital and at the forensic institute. Nevertheless, he became dependent upon the state hospital and did not want to leave. His speech was disorganized and difficult to follow. He believed that he was Jesus Christ. Alternately, and sometimes within minutes, he believed he was the devil. Ira's lability had an organic quality. His inveterate violence, sexual aggression, and mercurial, polarized delusions fluctuating without an ostensible precipitant from grandiose to self-diminishing made him fearsome. Staff dreaded contact with him, particularly if unaccompanied.

When he left the hospital, clinicians were required to visit him in his apartment, because of the nature of the rehabilitation program and the medication monitoring. Often a clinician had to be alone with him. When the clinician was a young female, she was at great risk of being sexually intimidated by his remarks, lewd staring, and excessive physical proximity or of being sexually molested. Such events were unpredictable. An easy solution would have been to send only male staff to his apartment or to provide only males when contacts had to be made with one unaccompanied case manager. However, such a solution was impractical because female case managers outnumbered males ten to one and many male patients had similar difficulties containing their sexual expression.

Of course, education and confrontation were provided routinely. Ira was repeatedly reminded not to touch or attempt to kiss staff. Clinicians were instructed about how to dress and behave and educated about the importance of insisting upon maintaining arms-length distance with all patients. This level of counseling is surely worth providing, but only helps some patients. Although Ira was able to repeat what he heard accurately, he could not retain these guidelines about staff–patient interactions. He was arrested many times for sexually assaulting female staff. Whether he had been arrested or not, Ira always seemed apologetic when confronted after these events.

He frequently asked his doctor if he could get some medicine to help him stop thinking so much about girls.

Male staff were also sexually assailed by Ira, but did not complain and discussed the situation only when asked. They were unwilling to press charges against Ira for sexually assaulting them. Though male staff said they were unafraid and not intimidated by Ira, there were not enough male staff to provide sufficient care for Ira to remain in the community. Female staff were afraid to visit him to help him with grooming, cooking skills, keeping his apartment clean, taking his medicine, and other critical aspects of self-care. The need for rehabilitation in his home was ongoing since Ira was not able to sustain his progress without considerable consistent support. Ira was destined to spend most of his time alone in his room hallucinating and in psychiatric hospitals because conventional neuroleptics only partially attenuated his symptoms. At last Clozaril became available for general use in the treatment of severe, medicine-resistant schizophrenia.

Ira the Pleasant

Considerable improvements in Ira's behavior and thinking were apparent within weeks of his beginning Clozaril. The first change, however, was unexpected and alarming. Ira became very taciturn, hardly speaking. He often became tearful and could not explain why. His appetite diminished, and he lost weight. He said that he belonged in hell. There was no obvious reason for this behavior. Clinicians' fascination with this carefree, superficial, and dangerous person's abrupt transition to a weeping and somber human was mingled with a sense of puzzlement. Why was Ira sad? He was no longer violent. His sexual behaviors were confined to ogling and staring. His brother was spending more time with him and was calling the center to say that Ira was better and to ask what else he could do to help him. Ira was washing himself, taking care of his roommate, who was not doing as well, and dressing very nicely, but did not want to eat or leave his apartment unless accompanied by a clinician. Yet he had become polite. He said "thank you" after many of his appointments. "Thank you" was not a phrase clinicians heard very often at an inner-city mental health center. He opened doors and stood aside for women he had formerly molested. Clinicians were giving Ira a great deal of attention and approval. One day, weeks after desipramine, an antidepressant, and group psychotherapy had been added to his treatment, Ira began to talk.

Ira's Unexpected Declaration

"I'm not Jesus Christ anymore. . . . I belong to Jesus Christ." Ira continued, "This medicine you're giving me . . . it's no good for me. . . . It's making me remember things I want to forget." He notified his therapy group of another dimension of his feeling: "Why are you giving me this medicine? It's making me feel so bad."

At other times Ira realized how much the medicine had helped him. His concentration had improved to the extent that the vocational rehabilitation program was considering him for a job at a time when paying positions for thinking-disabled people were too few and far between and at a premium. He was no longer paranoid. Ira "the terrible," a man of few comprehensible words, finally remembered, identified, and spoke of his memories.

Painful memories of being sexually molested by an uncle during his childhood emerged: "Yes, it was very humiliating." He became very despondent. "The medicine you're giving me is no good for me," he repeated several times.

Ira the Praiseworthy

He did it. Ira had reached a higher level of self-expression. He had moved beyond acting aggressively and in a disorganized

manner to verbalizing his memories and feelings in a safe
holding environment. Ira stopped crying. He placed his whole
interest in obtaining a job and did not feel the need to come to
group psychotherapy every other week. His remarks to staff
went as far as "I was thinking about you," and not further. It
was refreshing not to see Ira every other week or so with some
new problem stemming from the unsuitable enactment of
aggression or sexuality. He got a job potting plants in a
nursery. The job went so well that he extended his hours. We
did not see Ira for over six months. Knowing Ira as we did, no
news was good news.

After six months Ira returned to his group psychotherapy. He was not intrusive. He waited his turn to speak. He
looked at each group member who spoke, instead of putting
his head on the table, staring at the wall, or interrupting with
bizarre and irrelevant statements about Jesus Christ. He told a
group member who was complaining that her medicine made
her tired and was reporting that she had not taken it as
prescribed, "You should take your medicine . . . . That way it
will help you." Dottie, who was very noncompliant and
resistant to any intervention, listened to him: "I guess you're
right. I'll take it so I can get better." When someone asked him
about his job, Ira explained what he was doing. He spoke very
well. Ira appeared very pleased, rightly so, without a trace of
grandiosity.

Ira enjoyed music and weightlifting. No longer spending
time in jail and working at a paying job provided him extra
opportunities and money to enjoy his interests more fully.

DISCUSSION AND CONCLUSION: DID
PSYCHOTHERAPY HELP?

We anticipate that some readers will have the inevitable question of whether Henry, Lance, and Ira really needed psycho-

therapy. Would clozapine alone, slowly and over time, have helped them attain a healthy sense of self and an expanded capacity to work and relate to other people?

Health care costs are rising exponentially. Managed care companies are committed to controlling costs and can only survive the competition if they succeed in their mission. Mental health services are always most vulnerable to being excluded from receiving scarce resources as our evaluation of mental illness is still based upon consequences rather than causes and our diagnostic techniques have not generally made use of such high-tech modalities as blood tests and brain imaging that give numeric and visible value to illness and treatment. Administrators of mental health care programs of all kinds want to know whether medication, psychotherapy, or rehabilitation/case management alone could have brought about the same results. And they prefer concrete measurements or visualizable tests such as brain imaging as indicators of improvement. Clinical anecdotes speak poignantly of a person's quality of life, but carry little significance in our number-based world.

Yet, there are convincing improvements in various psychometric scales that affirm the extraordinary efficacy of clozapine and risperidone in reducing psychotic symptoms and increasing the quality of life. Pharmaceutical companies are paying great attention to quality of life scales and symptom rating scales in trying to discover and develop new medications.

Meanwhile, psychotherapists have generally relied more on the personal approach, measuring improvement by careful clinical observation and listening to the patient. With the added resource of case managers, we have the ability to observe patients in their usual daily life as well as in our office. We have presented four patients as an example of many action-driven people we have followed. We usually tend to put them in one category, as if they are all alike. We discovered, however, that while they shared some characteristics that were impossible to dismiss, they each had differences. They were able to define themselves further with the help of clozapine and psychotherapy and to find happiness each in his own unique way.

We find it impossible to believe that people who had improved significantly but were muddling along without a sense of purpose or direction for months would suddenly get their lives together in the ways we have described without psychotherapy. As soon as people have experienced sudden change after lifelong pervasive mental illness and institutionalization, they will most likely require serious focused effort to help raise their adjustment to the highest level possible, as well as opportunities to express themselves as distinctive and special people.

We are reminded of Kipling's words (1894): "Hah! The hooded Death has missed!"

10

Clara's Selves

And what about your dreams? the doctor one day asks me.
I tell him I do not dream.
I do not dare tell him about the dream I have every
night that terrifies me.

Alice Walker, *Possessing the Secret of Joy*

In Alice Walker's remarkable book, her protagonist Tashi has dreams of terror that she cannot reveal. She is from a culture in which female circumcision, the mutilation of young girls' genitals, is practiced. The haunting themes of the delusions of some patients sound like such dreams of terror as well. One patient in particular, Clara, has dreams and delusions of genital mutilation and threats that preoccupy much of her day. Are these delusions based in any actual experience? We do not know, and Clara does not tell us. Would it have mattered if we had asked such questions earlier in her illness? It may be too late to know.

We have observed a consistent improvement in patients' ability to control impulses while taking Clozaril. This seems to be true for patients whose impulses lead them to commit acts of violence and self-destructiveness, to abuse substances, and to engage in compulsive sexual behavior. Clinically, this effect is extremely important because as long as patients engage in impulsive and self-destructive behaviors, progress on other fronts is always limited. A reduction in impulsive behavior permits our patients to be more cognitively, interpersonally, and socially accessible. It makes it possible for them to develop and to receive more positive reactions from those around them.

A decrease in impulsive behavior also enables the clinician to look more closely at the patient as a whole and to consider issues that were of necessity set aside when impulsiveness was prominent. In this chapter we discuss a patient whose impulsiveness prior to taking Clozaril had so dominated her clinical picture that other considerations about her treatment needs could not be made. As she improved on Clozaril, other issues emerged.

Clara is a single white woman in her fifties, whose psychiatric history dates back over more than thirty years, most of them lived in psychiatric hospitals. Until she was discharged from a state hospital two years ago, she had been hospitalized almost continuously since her twenties. Clara has been diagnosed with schizophrenia, paranoid type, and historically her diagnosis has not been a point of controversy.

Clara was raised in a solidly middle-class household. Her developmental course was essentially normal until her father died when Clara was in her early teens. There are no clear reports of physical or sexual abuse, and Clara denies that abuse occurred. (An early medical record raises the question of abuse, but no further data were obtained.) Her first psychiatric hospitalization occurred when Clara was 17. Initially she received care from the best private psychiatric institutions in Connecticut, although with little apparent success. Starting in her twenties, Clara was treated in the state system. She lived in a state hospital continuously for fifteen years until her discharge at age 48.

Clara has never exhibited a formal thought disorder, nor does she complain of hearing voices. The primary characteristics of Clara's illness have been her delusions of sexual and physical violation, somatic hallucinations that this is occurring, and the agitation she feels in response.

Clara's response to Clozaril has been marked, but limited. On other, older neuroleptics she was assaultive to others and was delusional that she was being physically and sexually assaulted. On Clozaril Clara is more relaxed, no longer violent, less suicidal in ideation, and more capable of autonomous functioning. Yet, she still evidences a clear psychosis and still suffers from unusually florid and vivid persecutory delusions. However, she says she feels better on Clozaril and has been able to leave the hospital and live in a supervised apartment in the community for nearly two years.

After taking Clozaril for one month Clara moved from a hospital into a supervised group home in late 1993. Although her adjustment was difficult she has managed to remain in that home. She continues to believe that she is being attacked by "invisible penises" that fly through the air at her, raping her anally and vaginally, that machine guns have been strapped to her body along with grenades (also invisible), and that she is at risk of being forced into prostitution. Although the intensity of these beliefs seems muted since she has been on Clozaril, they remain her primary preoccupation.

The delusional content of Clara's illness has not been dulled by Clozaril, but she is quieter and in better control. Perhaps because she is less overtly combative, other symptoms have become the focus of more concentrated attention. Clara speaks of various selves. She describes them similarly to the way patients with dissociative identity disorder (DID) describe their parts: a "sexy" one, a "chaste" one, and others. These parts have names thath seem to derive from her name (Clarice, Lara, Clarabelle), a feature also noted among DID alters. Clara has been observed to space out and be unresponsive to staff, but she does not describe amnestic periods. And although she describes different identities and claims, for example, that Clarice is speaking rather than Clara, changes in her presentation have not been noted by others.

Clara was invited to join the Clozaril group, but she attended only sporadically over the course of two years. When she did attend, she would sit on the periphery, although her comments about others were always pertinent and lucid. Her comments about herself, in contrast, were usually focused on her delusions. She often excused herself during the group. Despite efforts to integrate her, Clara never seemed to experience herself as a member.

Clara also attended weekly individual psychotherapy sessions with a psychologist who was experienced in the treatment of DID. This psychotherapy was initiated both for purposes of clarifying Clara's diagnosis and because her team hoped that she might respond to a psychotherapeutic relationship in which her bizarre ideas were tolerated and with someone who would be attuned to dissociative experiences as they emerged. Although Clara attended psychotherapy sessions with some regularity and she claimed she enjoyed the meetings (indeed she was, if anything, overly grateful for her therapist's time), little distance from her persecutory beliefs developed nor was much clarity of diagnosis achieved. If anything, the clinician grew more perplexed about the dimensions of Clara's illness, which did not seem to fit neatly into either the dissociative or the schizophrenic spectrum. Clara terminated this therapy after two years, thanking the therapist profusely for her efforts and stating simply that she felt it was time to do other things.

SCHIZOPHRENIA AND DISSOCIATIVE IDENTITY DISORDER: DIFFERENTIAL DIAGNOSTIC ISSUES

The dissociative disorder literature suggests that some patients diagnosed with chronic schizophrenia may instead have a severe and chronic dissociative disorder. This error in diagnosis stems from the history of psychiatry, which until recently had largely disregarded dissociative disorders (Ellenberger 1970) and had instead attributed an array of symptoms exclusively to the psychotic disorders category (Kluft 1987). This section describes this historic diagnostic problem.

During the first half of this century, diagnostic convention followed Schneider's description of "first-rank symptoms" (FRS), which were generally considered pathognomonic of schizophrenia. These FRS symptoms include auditory hallucinations; feelings, thoughts, and actions experienced as intrusive or forced on the individual against his or her will; somatic passivity, perceived as a physiological influence from an external force; and thought withdrawal, insertion, broadcasting, and delusions. By 1973, Carpenter and colleagues (1973) documented that Schneiderian symptoms were not exclusive to schizophrenia, but rather occurred in a variety of psychotic illnesses. They cautioned, "Schneider's system for identifying schizophrenia, while highly discriminating, leads to significant diagnostic errors if FRSs are regarded as pathognomonic" (p. 847).

More precise descriptions of the characteristics of schizophrenia led to the distinction between positive and negative symptom syndromes (Kay et al. 1987). The Schneiderian FRS are entirely "positive", being the florid symptoms of delusions, hallucinations, and disorganized thinking. The negative symptoms are characterized by deficits in thinking, feeling, and social behavior, including blunted affect, passivity, and withdrawal (Kay et al. 1987). These symptoms are sometimes referred to as deficit symptoms. Carpenter and colleagues (1973) note incidences of positive FRS among patients diagnosed with schizophrenia, affective psychoses, neuroses, and character disorders. Kluft (1987) describes the frequency of first-rank (positive) symptoms among patients diagnosed with multiple personality disorder.

The observation that patients with multiple personality disorder (or, per the *DSM-IV*, dissociative identity disorder) frequently present with positive, "Schneiderian" symptoms has led to several reviews of the overlap among symptoms of schizophrenia and severe dissociative disorders (Ellason and Ross 1995, Fink and Golinkoff 1990, Ghadirian et al. 1985, Ross and Norton, 1988, Ross et al. 1994). This overlap raises several issues. First is the need to establish the correct diagnoses of patients who present with a set of symptoms conventionally considered psychotic. Presumably there are some cases in which patients with severe dissociative disorders have been misdiagnosed as schizophrenic due to the presence of Schneiderian first-rank symptoms.

Research supports the assumption of diagnostic confusion. Ross and colleagues (1990) have found that severely dissociative patients presented with more Schneiderian symptoms than did patients with schizophrenia. Ellason and Ross (1995) compare the frequency of reports of positive and negative symptoms among patients with schizophrenia and DID. In their research, patients with schizophrenia reported more negative symptoms than DID patients reported, but patients with DID reported more positive symptoms than did those with schizophrenia. Fink and Golinkoff (1990) note other symptoms that differentiate patients with DID from those with schizophrenia. Dissociative patients had more somatic symptoms, were more frequently severely depressed, exhibited more dissociative symptoms, and had more severe childhood trauma histories than did schizophrenics.

Thus there is a basis for the concern that some patients diagnosed with a severe and intractable schizophrenia may instead have a severe dissociative disorder. In addition, more complex diagnostic and treatment questions arise concerning patients who might suffer from comorbid psychotic and posttraumatic illnesses.

Why Were the Dissociative Disorders Ignored?

Stated most succinctly, the dissociative disorders seem to develop in the context of severe and prolonged childhood physical and/or sexual abuse (Kluft 1985, Ross 1989). But for many years, childhood abuse was simply not recognized as an aspect of the histories of many psychiatric patients. In consequence, the particular nature of the psychiatric consequences of abuse was not described.

Why was psychiatry blind to childhood abuse and its psychiatric consequences in adulthood? Several historians of psychiatry have reviewed this issue (Ellenberger 1970, van der Kolk and van der Hart 1989), and they describe the following sequence of events. Freud, one of the first modern thinkers in psychiatry, initially attributed much of the disordered behavior and thought that he encountered to inappropriate sexual stimulation suffered in childhood. As he came to theorize about the unconscious, however, Freud was persuaded to think increasingly about the developing child's fantasy life. In this process, he renounced the cause of neurosis as being actual abuse. He instead focused on his hypothesis that developing children naturally have sexual wishes about their parents (the Oedipus complex) and that the process of renunciation of this love leads to psychological maturity via development of the mature defensive process called repression. In essence, Freud stated that he had mistaken reports of infantile fantasy as statements of actual experience. "This shift in attention from the study of the effects of actual traumatic experiences to the psychology of repressed wishes and instincts marked the founding of psychoanalysis" (van der Kolk and van der Hart 1989, p. 1531).

Not until the 1970s did psychiatric researchers return to the investigation of the fact of childhood sexual abuse and its impact on the developing child. Since the mid-1980s research has established the frequency of childhood physical and sexual abuse among psychiatric patients (Beck and van der Kolk 1987, Carmen et al. 1984, Craine et al. 1988, den Herder and Redner 1991, Jacobson 1989, Muenzenmaier et al. 1993, Rose et al. 1991). There is a growing literature on the psychiatric consequences of childhood physical and sexual abuse (Cour-

tois 1988, Kluft 1985, 1990). These writers consistently describe disorders characterized by severe dissociative
symptoms as the consequence of childhood physical and
sexual abuse. For the community that treats the persistently
and severely mentally ill, recognition of abuse raises many
important issues, including the accuracy or adequacy of long-
held diagnoses and the completeness of treatment offered to
these patients.

DISCUSSION

So what is Clara's diagnosis? She has always been diagnosed
with schizophrenia, and indeed she has many symptoms of
that disorder. But she would seem to present some of the
problems addressed by the dissociative disorder literature. She
has flagrant positive, Schneiderian first-rank symptoms and
few negative symptoms. After thirty years of illness, many
schizophrenic patients are observed to burn out. In contrast,
and more like Clara, dissociative patients do not (Quimby et
al. 1993). She describes alters who she claims behave as DID
alters do, although such behavior has not been observed by her
clinical team. At times she may dissociate. She is preoccupied
with sexual and physical assault as are persons who have
experienced such assaults.

    Although the form of much of Clara's illness might fit the
description of exceptional dissociative symptoms, her distance
from accurate reality testing seems too great to accept her
disorder as purely dissociative. Inevitably, the illness with
which Clara presents today has been shaped by thirty years of
hospitalization. Elsewhere (Nasper and Smith 1995) we speculate that chronically hospitalized patients with dissociatve
illnesses might have learned to adapt their symptom picture to
an environment that only perceived experience through the
schizophrenic lens. The state hospital environment may have
shaped Clara to present her symptoms as more bizarre and

psychotic than was her original experience of them. Perhaps she has a severe schizophrenia. Or she may indeed have a comorbid psychosis and dissociative disorder, the result of an unidentified, hypothesized childhood trauma and her inherited biochemistry.

At this point in psychiatric history, diagnosis is almost entirely clinically derived: we make diagnoses based on a consensus derived from reviewing trends in the individual's history, current symptoms, and family history. The research on DID raises the possibility that we may be incorrectly grouping patients who exhibit similar symptoms under the diagnosis of schizophrenia. In addition, patients like Clara raise the possibility that some patients exhibit the loss of reality testing characteristic of schizophrenia along with the positive symptoms frequently found in dissociative disorders as well: perhaps these patients exhibit a comorbid dissociative disorder and schizophrenia.

PART III

Useful Ideas and Techniques for Psychotherapy with People Unexpectedly Recovering from Severe, Prolonged Psychosis

11

Psychotherapy with Patients Recovering from Years of Psychosis

Dionysus had turned up in the role of Unknown Guest in the house of an old Attican gardener, Icarius, who lived with his daughter Erigone and loved to plant new types of trees. His house was a poor one. All the same, he welcomed the Stranger with the same gesture with which Abraham welcomed the angel, by keeping a place in his mind empty and ready for his guest. It was from that gesture that every other gift would derive.

Roberto Calasso, *The Marriage of Cadmus and Harmony*

SOME THOUGHTS ABOUT THE NEED FOR PSYCHOTHERAPY

In the late 1980s treatment of severely disturbed psychiatric patients emphasized medications and intensive case management approaches. It was hoped that new biological interventions alone would cure psychiatric illness and that all severely disturbed patients needed was assurance that they received their medications and had a modicum of organization in their lives. The benefit of this emphasis was clear: it was our experience that intensive case management programs ensured that patients received the medications and day-to-day assistance they needed, resulting in a marked reduction in inpatient hospitalizations.

On the other hand, this perspective led to a neglect of the patient's internal mental life—his or her feelings, motivation, and point of view. Clinicians who were hired to be case managers sometimes found themselves without tools to motivate patients, to asssist them to change attitudes or behaviors, or to leave chronically abusive home situations, because these clinicians had not been trained to make such interventions. In addition, the concrete daily demands of their case management tasks occupied all of their energies. Psychotherapy was disparaged, and those who had been trained as psychotherapists often felt irrelevant to the intensive case management programs. As a consequence, exploration and acknowledgment of motivation, feelings, and point of view were far too often excluded from the treatment of the most severely disturbed, as though these patients lacked an internal mental life that was intimately involved with their illness and their psychosocial adjustment. Clinicians had not figured out ways to adapt their understanding of the mental life to the new types of treatment interventions, and many felt the irrelevance of the psychotherapeutic perspective.

One of the unfortunate consequences of this shift in emphasis was the implication that helping patients explore or understand their internal life—the life of private thoughts, emotions, fantasies, and wishes—was not useful in the treatment of severely disturbed patients. The disparagement of psychotherapy was supported by economic pressures, since staff who were trained to think about the internal mental life were generally professionally trained and therefore more expensive than nonprofessionally trained case managers. This is not to argue that the support provided through intensive case management was not necessary. However, neglect of a perspective that included awareness of the patient's internal world meant that our understanding of our patients was significantly limited.

Clozaril introduced a need to rethink our treatment of chronically ill patients. The introduction of a new biological agent provoked enormous psychological changes in our patients, and adjustment to these changes did not seem to be automatic. We had to consider psychological interventions to assist in this adjustment.

Perhaps the sequence of events described above was attributable in part to the limits of the traditional neuroleptics. Traditional neuroleptics tend to target the positive symptoms of schizophrenia, and patients often continue to have significant negative symptoms: flattened affect, little motivation, apathy, and a kind of interpersonal dullness. In addition, because they often suffer disfiguring movement disorders, they may withdraw socially since they feel shame and discomfort about the way they look. The most striking positive outcome with Clozaril has been the reduction of both negative and positive symptoms. Somebody comes home when Clozaril is successful. Patients become more spontaneous, more engaged, and more lively as human beings. The medication seems to permit the restoration of a more accessible sense of self. But with that enhanced sense of self comes a wide range of thoughts and feelings that presents enormous challenges to some patients.

A BRIEF BACKGROUND TO THE PSYCHOTHERAPY GROUP

When Clozaril was originally prescribed in 1991, patients were seen biweekly in a medication monitoring group. After several months, many exhibited significant symptomatic improvement, but few had made significant changes in their lives. Patients who had been chronically agitated, grossly psychotic, or plagued with negative symptoms seemed better, and objective measures supported this observation. Clinicians wondered how to motivate patients to function better.

We were struck that some patients had apparent difficulty tolerating their improvement. This problem seemed especially poignant for Zack, described in detail in Chapter 4, whose marked improvement made his frequent refusal of medication difficult to understand. The most compelling explanation of his choice seemed to be that Zack could not bear the adjustment demanded by his change. Zack and others floundered despite their improved mental status. It was apparent that a successful biological intervention was not enough and that our patients needed a new dimension in their treatment. After the medication group had been meeting for two years, the Clozaril psychotherapy group developed to meet this need.

THE MEDICATION GROUP

The purpose of the Clozaril medication group was to monitor the symptoms and side effects of Clozaril and to provide new prescriptions. There were enough patients on Clozaril that having just one group was unwieldy. Therefore the group met on alternating weeks; its composition was largely dictated by when case managers could bring their patients to the meetings.

The group adhered to few psychotherapy group norms. The prescribing psychiatrist was the central figure and the central focus of communication. Case managers and patients interacted primarily with the doctor to discuss the recent functioning of individual patients.

A great strength of the group, which was striking even to the new observer, was that patients experienced it as a safe holding environment. They attended regularly, they wanted the psychiatrist's attention, and they seemed to feel comfortable and supported by her. This environment served as the base for a more exploratory group; without it, we would not have been able to address some of the difficult issues that later arose.

On the other hand, there were significant problems in the process. There was little intragroup relating. Group norms included an open flow of patients and staff in and out of the room. Side conversations were accepted and initiated by both patients and staff. An individual patient's absence was not a group concern, nor was an individual patient's return particularly noted or acknowledged.

These norms were consistent with the long-term experience of the patients in the group. Their individual lives had become defined by their identity as mental patient. This role implied little appreciation of their individuality, little right to privacy, little recognition of the value of what the individual patient had to say. That the group functioned in a way that was socially chaotic and disrespectful of all participants was obvious to any new observer. However, its functioning represented a norm often characteristic of staff interactions with chronic psychiatric patients. It was as though everyone had tacitly agreed to assume that no one noticed or was bothered by people coming and going, that patients were not interested in what other patients had to say, and that a patient's view of him- or herself was not of particular weight in making treatment decisions. Such behavioral norms could not foster independence of thought or action because they demonstrated so little respect for the patients' thoughts and actions.

The Negative Impact of Negative Symptoms

These behavioral norms may become accepted by staff and patients alike because patients' negative symptoms may make them seem oblivious to their surroundings. On recovery, however, many patients report an awareness of their experiences from periods when they may have appeared out of touch. A passive response to disrespectful treatment is often characteristic of people with poor self-esteem, and this may also contribute to the development of a treatment atmosphere in which there is little appreciation for the individuality of the patient. It also seems possible that we altered the atmosphere in response to the patients' improved cognitive abilities. As they improved we were able to identify more directly with them and could no longer permit ourselves to treat them with less consideration.

THE PSYCHOTHERAPY GROUP

Goals

The primary goal of the psychotherapy group was to assist patients to identify and accept a new sense of self. Through group discussions we helped participants (1) become more aware of and name their feelings, clarify their opinions, and notice that disagreement was possible and tolerable; (2) reflect on the experience of extended hospitalization and how living in the community differed from it; (3) challenge rigid ideas about themselves, others, and the nature of reality; (4) enhance their flexibility of thought to reduce isolation and loneliness; and (5) identify and articulate goals. We wanted the participants to feel that their individuality was valued and validated. We hoped that each member would enjoy the group meetings and would leave with an enhanced sense of self-worth and a developed capacity and comfort in social interactions. Ultimately we hoped that these gains would generalize to their relationships within the community at large.

Accomplishing the Goals

To work toward these goals for the group, we took a stance similar to that described by Dewald (1994). Our intent was to be ego-supportive and reality based in order to facilitate interpersonal communication and an honest appraisal of self. We avoided all but the most gentle confrontations and of necessity tolerated psychotic wanderings. While we generally focused on the present, the past was acknowledged to be relevant. For example, mention of past abuse became the opportunity for education about its ongoing psychological consequences. When it seemed helpful, we explicitly related early self-concept and expectations to the way individuals felt about their current capabilities.

We proceeded with several unarticulated premises in the development of these interventions. Foremost was an assumption that the essence of promoting psychological development was contained in the formation of a reliable, committed therapeutic relationship. In this relationship, the therapist's goal was to facilitate the patient's self-knowledge through enhancing their capacity to observe and reflect on their experience and to realistically assess their perceptions. This goal could be furthered through a variety of methods: education, discussion, and even interpretation of motives or defenses if the patient could tolerate and use such intervention. In addition, the therapist came to the relationship informed about normal defenses and psychotic thought processes. The psychotherapeutic approach was informed by psychoanalytic concepts, even if the techniques were eclectic and pragmatically determined. Inevitable psychological events such as transference, countertransference, projection, displacement, and so on were recognized by the therapists, but often they were not interpreted to the patient.

To illustrate when we did and did not interpret the patients' unconscious process, we use two examples involving

Paula. Paula had just begun to respond to Clozaril, and the most striking initial impact of her recovery was a significant reduction of her paranoia. Nonetheless, when threatened, Paula's usual stance was anger. On one occasion a few months after the feelings group started, Paula was angry about something. We raised the possibility that, in addition to being angry, perhaps she was hurt. Paula recognized herself in this description and seemed relieved and comforted that her experience was recognized. Earlier on she probably would have defensively rejected this elaboration of her feeling state. At this point, however, she was able to use it to expand her awareness of the emotional dimensions of her experience.

In contrast, at a later group it began to emerge that Paula had a crush on one of the group leaders. Her medical record indicated that at one time she had questions about her sexual orientation. But her recent expressions had made clear that she was anxious about any erotic expression and in addition was somewhat (albeit defensively) homophobic. We therefore noted to ourselves her transferential feelings but did not mention these observations in group. To have done so explicitly would have humiliated and disorganized her. Our goal was to maintain and support her defensive structure, not to explore her erotic fantasy. Were she to have consciously raised these issues, however, we would have welcomed their discussion. By "keeping a place in [our] mind empty and ready for [our] guest" (Calasso 1993, p. 37), we hoped that our patients would also be permitted to reveal themselves to us, to themselves, and to each other.

Norms

We elected not to structure the group with regard to the content of the discussion. But we did try to structure the form of the group in these ways: meeting at a set time, discouraging side conversations, permitting only one person to talk at a

time, and encouraging members to talk with one another
rather than to or through the therapists. We tried to acknowledge members' absences, to comment on their whereabouts,
and to acknowledge their return.

Interestingly, some patients found this concern on others' behalf intrusive. When we announced to the group that
Zack had been rehospitalized, the group met this news ambi-
valently. Initially, Dan felt it was none of our business: "He
can handle himself. He's very adequate. If he's in the hospital
we shouldn't miss him."

Others were troubled, feeling that to discuss people in
their absence violated their privacy. On the other hand, the
fact that Zack's functioning had declined had been noticed.
One member empathized with Zack's point of view: "It could
be vice versa, too. He could be saying, 'I wonder what's going
on in the group.' "

Content

When it was decided that the medication group needed a more
psychotherapeutic dimension, a psychologist was invited to
join the group. Initially, she raised various pointed questions
about the members' adjustment to Clozaril. The group members attempted to answer her, but the resulting discussion bore
more resemblance to a stilted interview than to a psychotherapy group.

It was soon apparent that for the group to be meaningful
to the participants, the content needed to vary as natural
conversation does. Rather than directing the content, we
learned to amplify themes spontaneously introduced by the
patients. A group member's observation of artwork in our
room instigated a discussion of past and present creative out-
lets of the members, which yielded important information
about the patients' identities prior to their illness. One group
member, who had been a competitive skater from a family of

skaters, contributed facts about local sports history. This expanded our view of this person, her past, and her potential and
clarified and raised our expectations of what she might contribute to the group.

Members

From among the patients on Clozaril a cohort was selected
that had demonstrated increased social interaction and interest
in others. These members were a core group, but others joined
for periods of time or kept a peripheral membership. Patients
who have expressed an interest in the group have been welcomed, and members have been excluded only for disruptive
behavior.

Staff membership in the group could also be divided into
core and peripheral. The cotherapists came consistently, as did
one case manager. The agency chaplain joined the group for
several months, and during that time she was an active member. Nursing staff from the treatment team attended more
sporadically, but eventually one nurse attended as a regular
group member.

Process

The process and the content of meetings have changed over
time much in the ways one would expect in any psychotherapy group. Patients direct their discussion to one another
much more than they did in the beginning; the relative weight
given to remarks by the leaders seems diminished as the
importance of peer interaction has increased. Members are
significantly more interested in one another than they were
initially, demonstrated by ten-minute discussions in which an
individual's issues will be everyone's focus of questions and
comments. Topics flow spontaneously, and the group no
longer relies on the staff leaders to get the discussion going.

The atmosphere of the group is more relaxed. Warm exchanges among members are surprisingly frequent events. A touching interchange that occurred while Zack was still in the group is illustrative. Zack was feeling pervasively sad about his life and commented that he wanted to "make up for lost time." Lannie comforted Zack with the observation, "You're a good man," to which Zack responded, "I wish I could have you as my father."

The clinicians use themselves and their life experiences to model aspects of coming to know and accept ourselves. We do this with prudence, restricting our self-disclosure to topics that have emerged from the patients' discussion, and where the self-disclosure serves to normalize their experience. We recognize several dangers in self-disclosure, including overwhelming the patients with information and concerns about their treaters or ending up using the group's time for personal ventilation. We have tried to avoid these risks. At the same time, illustrating how staff cope with interpersonal and internal dilemmas seems useful to some patients.

In December 1993 we found ourselves talking about the then-anticipated Haiti invasion. Billy said that he was grateful that Sean, his case manager, who is also in the Army Reserves, had not gone to Operation Desert Storm. When Sean asked why, Billy replied, "Because I like you." Sean was embarrassed and tried to change the subject. This provided an opportunity to explore why someone so obviously likable might be made uncomfortable by an expression of affection. With Sean's permission, we tried to elicit the reason for his discomfort, although it was apparent that this was hard for him to put into words. Our purpose through this interchange was to illustrate that a difficulty commonly experienced by the group members might be familiar to the staff as well. We have several goals in this type of intervention. It seems important to acknowledge that all of us function on a continuum, with areas of strength and weakness. It also is important to counter the fantasy that staff have solved all the problems in their lives.

Finally, we make the point that life without psychosis does not mean life without struggles and adjustments.

Topics

The group has addressed a wide range of subjects, all of them common to psychotherapy groups. The topics include relationships with parents, wishes for romantic relationships, anxiety about parental mortality, actual losses, work, conflicted feelings about illness and medications, good times and bad times, regrets, disappointments, wishes, hopes and dreams. We encourage all subjects, especially the ones that our patients tend to censor for themselves. In our experience, they seem most reluctant to explore their wishes and hopes for the future. We approach them holding the dialectic of acceptance and change: acceptance of the painful limits that have been part of their lives and encouragement of the striving for change and hope that can also be part of their lives. As stated earlier, with time the group members have initiated discussion and interchange with one another much more than was true at the beginning. They also take on the encouragement and support of each other.

CONCLUSION

In this chapter we have explored some aspects of doing a psychotherapy group with people who were recovering from years of psychosis. The psychotherapy we do involves a mix of exploration, support, assistance in reality testing, psychoeducation, and cheerleading. Over the course of our group, members have improved very significantly. Most strikingly, people who were initially irritable, delusional, thought disordered, and paranoid came alive, becoming articulate and more self-assured. They have improved their self-care, ceased abusing substances, and thought clearly and more empathically about one another. It is also clear that "recovery" is a risky word. Some of the patients who have been taken off Clozaril for various reasons quickly became floridly psychotic again.

All life issues, of course, were not solved by Clozaril. For some, the improvements presented new challenges that were met with mixtures of avoidance, anxiety and delight. For a few, the challenges of such radical improvement have as yet been intolerable, and they have chosen to discontinue Clozaril.

12

Before, During, and After Clozaril

Epimetheus had in his house a jar, in which were kept certain noxious articles. . . . Pandora was seized with an eager curiosity to know what this jar contained; and one day she slipped off the cover and looked in. Forthwith there escaped a multitude of plagues for hapless man—such as gout, rheumatism and colic for his body, and envy, spite and revenge for his mind—and scattered themselves far and wide. Pandora hastened to replace the lid! but, alas! the whole contents of the jar had escaped, one thing only excepted, which lay at the bottom, and that was hope.

Thomas Bulfinch, *The Age of Fable*

In preceding chapters we have presented many sad stories of disrupted lives, fragmented families, irreclaimable relationships, lost youth, and years of humiliating mental illness. Our stories are about the multitude of plagues that strike hapless human minds, plagues that override envy, spite, and revenge. Pestilence that brings appalling distortions in human thinking and behavior. Madness. Lunacy. Insanity. Derangement. All of these powerful words speak of formidable suffering. While all humans suffer, some seem to experience suffering to a greater extent than others. We have not yet attempted to explain why some people seem to suffer more than others or why some may have hope while others appear to have lost it. However, in this chapter, we describe some valuable insights offered by the allegory of Pandora into the stigma of illness and the reasons why good treatments for mental illness were so slow to develop.

The fable of Pandora attempts to explain how and why humanity was punished with the scourge of physical and mental illness. In one version Bulfinch tells us that Prometheus and his brother discovered fire in heaven. They then offered it to humanity to use and enjoy. Incensed, Jupiter created Pandora. He sent her to punish Prometheus and his brother for their presumption in taking fire from heaven, and to punish humanity for accepting the gift.

In our moments of rational thought we do not believe in Pandora or her indiscretion, just as we do not believe in Santa Claus. We view the punishment of women for inquisitiveness as reprehensible. And so we do not buy the opinion that humanity should be punished for achieving or benefiting from ground-breaking discoveries.

An interesting discrepancy exists between the rational and irrational. We live centuries after the Age of Reason at a time when civilized and logical thinking has attained refinement and has become widespread (sometimes). Curiosity is now touted as a virtue and recognized as a quality that may lead to momentous discoveries or further learning. Originators of new discoveries or pioneers of new ways of thinking are often praised and given Nobel prizes. Feminist thinking has debunked the notion that women should be punished or blamed for their curiosity or for seeking knowledge. Yet, despite feminism and other movements that have refined and revolutionized human thinking, humans continue to harbor and unabashedly promote archaic thinking.

RELEVANCE OF NONRATIONAL THINKING

Influential material from nonrational thinking often propels rational thinking and behavior unbeknown to us. Myth and fable are derivatives of the midbrain as well as many other brain structures, and are largely unconscious. Traversing cultural boundaries, they are widely available tools or opportunities to gain access to the resources of the unconscious. Many such tales are cross-breeds that convey similar ubiquitous themes. The similarity of the story of Adam and Eve's presumption in satisfying their desire for knowledge to the myth of Pandora is striking. Both resulted in punishment that unleashed sickness upon humanity.

People maintain a fascination with myth. Thinking about mental illness is influenced by nonrational thought, as well as by myths and fables.

Other culturally pervasive methods of communicating with the nonrational and the areas of the brain from which derive myths and dream states are the use of certain drugs (cocaine, marijuana, mescaline, peyote, LSD), hypnosis, particular forms of prayer, and controlled starvation (fasting). Learning to do business with the nonrational seems to be very important to humans. Freud is probably one of the best-known exponents of connecting to the unconscious through dreams and free association, thereby understanding and modulating it. The nonrational is also a fundamental source of creativity. Artists, musicians, poets, playwrights, discoverers and inventors of new things, humorists and comedians, and people interested in falling and staying in love all need to make contact with the nonrational for the inventive juices to flow.

Our point is to highlight the extent to which rational thinking about mental suffering has been colored by nonrational thought, beliefs, and myths. Mental illness seems especially twisted into a tangle of negative assumptions that have been impervious to many astonishing developments in understanding the neurophysiology of thinking and the neuropathology of mental illness.

BAD THINGS HAPPEN TO BAD PEOPLE

One common assumption, whether conscious or not, is that if misfortune happens, such as becoming mentally ill, the unlucky person must deserve it. Our mythology is replete with vivid and awesome stories of wrongdoing followed by retribution. Pandora is but one of them. According to one account, Pandora herself is a punishment. We discover from these rich and spellbinding stories that the notion of bad is very broad. Curiosity is bad. Disobedience is bad. Defining oneself as separate from parents is rebellious or treasonous. Trying new things is bad. Accepting gifts from Greeks is bad. The punishments, while having remarkable vitality and richness, are extreme and generally merciless. They can continue throughout a lifetime or for several generations; they can cause a person to blind himself or go mad.

Religion is another source of the tenet that bad things only happen to bad people. The adaptive value of this belief is easy to discern. People should not be bad; they should be good. If they are bad they will suffer consequences. If they don't want to endure retribution, they can find the means to stop or prevent being bad. This way of looking at life is simplistic but encouraging. The mesencephalon likes "simple."

In addition to the unconscious and the influence of religion, another buttress of the notion that bad things happen to bad people is the literature about the causes of mental illness.

A BRIEF HISTORY OF THEORIES OF THE CAUSES OF MENTAL ILLNESS

Magicians, poets, priests, nuns, kings, teachers, physicians, soothsayers, and fortune tellers, to name but a few, have bought into, promoted, and often profited from the idea that bad things befall defective, disobedient, harmful, immoral, inferior, substandard people. The converse of this view is that good things happen to obedient, virtuous, genuine, honest, and superior people.

Centuries went by before society had a clue that things are not as they seem. We do not know what raised societal awareness of the observation that good people also succumb to harm, pain, or illness or that bad people can escape those fates. However, deeply driven notions of mental illness have lingered. There continues to be a primitive cultural picture of madness, that people who lost their minds must have deserved their misfortune through some wrongdoing or mistake. Such views have hampered scientific discoveries about chemical imbalances in the central nervous system and their effect on mental illness. Like Pandora, the mentally ill or their family must have exhibited curiosity, greed for knowledge of the unknown, or espoused nonconformist ideas and someone had to be punished.

In some cultures, the group from which the lapse occurred must pay the consequences by sacrificing a victim, a member of the group, usually the proximate cause of the trouble or a politically unfavored person. The person afflicted by mental illness need not therefore be the guilty one. In Western culture, however, there is an emphasis on individual responsibility. The person who made the mistake has to be discovered and punished. Therefore, if you go mad in America, it is your fault, and you must suffer the consequences.

Authors of psychiatric literature of past epochs seem to reflect general societal views and values whether or not they are predicated on recently available factual information. The filtering down of knowledge to inform societal values takes a long time. Will societal attitudes and mores about mental illness ever completely absorb the discoveries of the past fifty years about the neuropathology and chemistry of mental illness? We are optimistic that they will. Yet we know there are other problems associated with the blossoming field of brain neuroscience.

BIAS TOWARD PSYCHIATRIC ILLNESS

Another problem besieging brain neuroscience and psychology has been the lack of technological devices to study delicate structures and molecular processes within the central nervous system as well as within other organs. For decades, evaluations of mental illness have lagged behind the rest of medicine and were predicated solely upon the effects and consequences of insanity rather than its causes. The lack of opportunity to investigate the actual origins of mental illness left doctors and society in the dark and was no doubt also responsible for the lower credibility accorded to psychiatric and psychological evaluation. Thus, the blaming of people and/or their family for the outcome of sickness of the mind and failure to respond to treatment by getting well has lingered. Scoping genetic structure; such brain imaging modalities as magnetic resonance imaging (MRI) and positron emission tomography (PET); and the development of refined, focused, and reliable tests and questionnaires to measure various aspects of the disturbances of thinking and feelings have given us reason to think there can be a new outlook on the comprehension of mental illness in society.

STABLE AND BASELINE

The treatment of persistent psychosis has entered an age of reason, when treatments beyond chaining people in dungeons, seclusion rooms, ice baths, insulin coma, electroconvulsive therapy, and lobotomy were developed. Such drugs as lithium and chlorpromazine (Thorazine) enabled patients to be stabilized for intervals long enough to allow discharge from the hospital. For some, the stability was sufficient to allow continuation of treatment in their hometown, with infrequent decompensation or rehospitalization. Such people were treatment sensitive, received substantial benefit from medication, and may never have required treatment in state hospitals.

While the controversy may still continue, there are strong proponents for the view that people with true schizophrenia (sometimes called core or nuclear schizophrenia) inevitably drift downward, losing the ability to work, insurance benefits, and family support, and end up relying on state facilities of mental health care for their treatment. This idea is concordant with the observation that many patients with schizophrenia treated in state hospitals and community mental health centers do not sustain a complete remission from their symptoms. The label of having residual symptoms is often used to capture their clinical outcome. However, the word "residual" minimizes the intensity of the lingering symptoms and degree of disability. The phrases "treatment refractory" or "incomplete remission" more accurately capture the amount of remaining illness, despite the patient's being stabilized. Indeed, the stabilized patient may not actually be stable in what little remission he or she has received from conventional treatment, but rather may be unstably-stable or stably-unstable.

What stabilized often really means is that the patient is not bothering us (the clinicians). When we are not notified of their suffering in dramatic ways or crisis mode, we often assume they are not suffering. The unstably-stable can muddle along for months in and out of intense symptoms, but are too disabled to support themselves before a more profound crisis precipitates decompensation. The stably-unstable muddle along with continuous and slow worsening of acute and subacute symptoms, eventually superseding our thresholds for illness. When they transcend our symptom threshold—in other words, bother us—they are thereby considered decompensated or no longer at baseline.

It is clear that, for many decades, the term *baseline* did not refer to a patient's premorbid (preschizophrenia) status, but to a stably disabled, noncrisis mode of being. Many people who were disabled mainly by negative symptoms of psychosis were considered baseline or stable, though they could not work or take care of themselves.

HOPE

Webster's Encyclopedic Unabridged Dictionary of the English Language (1989) defines hope as, "the feeling that what is desired is also possible, or that events may turn out for the best" (p. 683).

An example of hope is the feeling that people whose mental illness is treatment resistant or only partially relieved by conventional medication can do better. The hope that the desired improvement is also possible through a reduction in symptoms has been rekindled by new antipsychotic medication. After a twenty-year latency, new medications in development have finally become available for general use and have extraordinary efficacy in the treatment of formerly treatment-refractory symptoms. Stability and baseline can no longer be considered satisfactory treatment outcomes. It is necessary to enlarge those concepts, encompass humane and broadened aspirations. Enriched social, cognitive, and vocational functioning; diminished suicide rates and dangerousness to others; and reduction in substance abuse can now be confidently offered to almost all people suffering from mental illness, even though they may have been warehoused in asylums and given up as unable to accomplish further improvements. What is desired is possible.

GIVING SHAPE TO THE INVISIBLE WORLD

Will new medications put psychotherapists, case managers, and clinicians other than psychopharmacologists out of business? We think not. The experience of mental illness is dehumanizing. It is difficult to imagine that the sudden diminution of symptoms could automatically facilitate the complex leap of becoming part of a human community. This is rarely possible while patients are intensely cognitively compromised by deficit symptoms. Capturing a sense of self that goes beyond being a schizophrenic is more likely to ensue with psychotherapy. Offering people psychotherapy who have suddenly recovered from severe lifelong mental illness is critical, integral, and indispensable.

THE "MAD" NEUROTRANSMITTERS AND RECEPTORS

As more is learned about the biochemistry and neuropathology of mental illness, new medications are being designed and developed. The development process takes many years and the intensive labor of many people. After favorable results in bench research (yes, with rodents and primates), the new drugs must be tested in trials with people (clinical trials with the other branch of the primate tree) and must appear promising for better relief of the symptoms of psychosis. The new medicines also seem to be safer for patients than existing medications in clinical trials. The designer drugs are not just clones of Clozaril or Clozaril "wannabes." The new drugs are cultivated through major and carefully managed clinical trials.

The new medications are made up of molecules that attempt to affect pre- and postsynaptic membranes at the cellular level. Blocking critical serotonergic receptors (5HT-2 and HT1c) and achieving a better balance of dopamine receptor occupancy are currently considered critical in effecting better symptom remission with fewer side effects. There are many contenders for the clean (free of side effects) broad-spectrum, high-power, fail-safe antipsychotic.

The Leaders of the Pack, for Those Who Want to Know

Risperidone, olanzapine, ziprasidone, sertindole, and seroquel are a few of the new medications with new blends of receptor-blocking properties that seem to be outperforming conventional neuroleptics with fewer side effects. Unlike Clozaril, there have been no cases of suppression of the bone marrow's production of white blood cells. Therefore, the inconvenience of a weekly white blood cell count and the danger of an undetected reduction in white blood cells are eliminated. Pharmaceutical companies and clinicians hope that the efficacy of these new medications can measure up to Clozaril at least for some patients, though Clozaril is a tough act to follow. We describe each new and promising medication individually.

The Position and Importance of Risperidone

Risperidone (Risperdal) was released for general prescription use for the treatment of schizophrenia in 1993. It is the only one of the new drugs (novel antipsychotics) that is currently available outside a research study. It does not have as good a clinical track record as clozapine for people who are severely mentally ill. However, without question risperidone has dramatically reduced symptoms and improved the quality of life of many seriously ill people who have received only partial relief from standard antipsychotics. We have no way yet of identifying who will be most likely to benefit from it. The response of a patient to Clozaril seems to have no predictive value.

Risperidone has unique properties. The risk of developing abnormal movements at doses of 6 mg/day (or less) is diminished. There is no risk of bone marrow suppression or lowering the white blood cell count. Awakenings from lifelong mental illness have already occurred and more can be expected. Several of the people in our psychotherapy group who recovered dramatically from severe and lifelong mental illness while taking Clozaril needed to switch their medication to risperidone. Some of them continued to progress just as well after six months or more of risperidone treatment.

Olanzapine, the "Clean" Clozaril?

Olanzapine wants to be the clean Clozaril. Not that Clozaril is dirty but it does have a potentially fatal side effect. Clozaril can also cause some uncomfortable side effects such as weight gain, sedation, and drooling, although these disappear over a period of 3–12 months for most people. There is a greater potential for developing seizures while taking Clozaril, though we have not seen this adverse effect as frequently as reported in the literature. It would be a great advantage for a medication to be as effective as Clozaril for the treatment of persistent disabling mental illness without its possible effects on bone marrow (white blood cell problems).

Olanzapine is currently available only to patients who are enrolled in carefully performed studies (clinical trials). Because the number of patients taking olanzapine relative to clozapine and risperidone is small and all the collected data have not been made generally available, its actual risk/benefit profile is not certain. A combination of clinical study experience at our center and rumors circulating about olanzapine suggest that it is a winner. It is clearly a leading contender for a position next to Clozaril for effectiveness and above Clozaril for safety.

Ziprasidone, the Sexy Antipsychotic?

While the jury is still out on this new medication, ziprasidone is looking very good in clinical studies. In our experience it has a curious sexual effect. Many conventional antipsychotics seem to suppress sexual interest in partner sex. Clozapine and risperidone seem to increase patients' interest in dating, but the actual procedures around getting a date are slow to follow the interest.

Ben, a man who had spent many years of his life on the chronic units of state hospitals, had not expressed any interest in partner sex in many years, even while taking clozapine. Though he identified himself as heterosexual, he had never dated or had sex with a woman, and he professed to have arousing sexual fantasies only about men. During his treatment with ziprasidone in a clinical study at our center, his psychiatrist paged the clinical investigator of the study to report that Ben was following women around the unit and into their bedrooms. He was also observed trying to kiss and fondle them. Ziprasidone may be more effective in addressing the symptoms of low interest in partner sex and lack of confidence in the ability to carry the process forward.

The Two Promising S's

Sertindole and seroquel are both promising contenders for a position alongside clozapine. They are only presently available to patients who participate in clinical studies. Their effectiveness and safety seem to be very good. Reports of sudden relief of years of madness have not been published, but such accounts are usually withheld until a medication is nearer to FDA approval for general availability.

SIGNIFICANT RECOVERY DESPITE PERSISTENT SYMPTOMS

The literature on rehabilitation abounds in discussions about the importance of having a life despite restrictions imposed by persistent symptoms. Certainly this may be possible for some people. But our clinical experience is that for many others, having a satisfactory life while continuing to experience severe symptoms has been hard to achieve. Our central argument has been that until the recent development of improved medication, significant recovery was impossible for many patients afflicted by lifelong severe and relentless positive and negative symptoms of psychosis. We are aware that many patients had been warehoused in state hospitals. The existing rich resources of assertive case management and vocational/social rehabilitation were sufficient to facilitate improvement in symptoms, function, and the self-concept of these people. They were thereby able to accomplish a significant recovery. However, when cognition is so gravely compromised as in many of our patients, that person's experience is so internally referenced that any relationship-facilitated rehabilitation (or psychotherapy) will be largely unsuccessful. Negative symptoms and extreme positive symptoms of psychosis are dehumanizing and for the most part make recovery inaccessible to that person until superior medication to relieve those symptoms is provided.

Leroy Spaniol (1995) presented some of his thinking about the symptoms of mental illness and recovery at the Janssen Pharmaceutica CNS Roundtable. His ideas are relevant and worth reviewing. Spaniol regards recovery as a common human experience. We are all recovering from some tragedy or trauma such as the death of a loved one, divorce, or the loss of hopes and dreams we couldn't achieve. He emphasizes the importance of having an internal sense of self despite or separate from external events. Life experiences are disconnected by trauma. Working on an internal sense of self that places external events in perspective is of vital importance. The sense of self is based on acting in our own interest, work, and finding role models. Spaniol contrasts the old notion of recovery with evolving notions. The previous view of recovery was that a patient would get better (free of symptoms), feel fine, not require medication or other ongoing treatment, and

experience a "complete" recovery. Such thinking is not realistic for people who have been traumatized by persistent
mental illness. Modern thinking about recovery emphasizes
the need to lead a full life with limitations, medication, and
symptoms. The outcome of the treatment of symptoms need
not be confused with a person's functional illness, that is, the
fullness of life that the person can experience.

Spaniol's thinking is compelling. However, medication
that can truly effect adequate symptom relief, even though not
curative (residual symptoms often persist), was a necessary
component for some of the gravely mentally ill to be empow-
ered to enter meaningful recovery. We acknowledge that
psychotherapy is expensive to provide. We know that managed care wants to get rid of relationship-mediated treatment.
We are also aware that we cannot identify who among our
symptomatically improved patients progressed in their recovery because of psychotherapy and would not have had the
same positive outcome had expensive and in some cases
lengthy psychotherapy not been provided.

People who have experienced sudden dramatic symptom
relief and who are just muddling along or floundering are
profoundly confused and unable to make use of their new lease
on a fulfilling life. Because of the thoroughly dehumanizing
experience of madness, we feel that psychotherapy should be
routinely offered in addition to case management and rehabilitation.

How much psychotherapy should be supplied, or when
should treatment end? Psychotherapy should be offered until
the patient demonstrates a readiness and ability to move forward with his or her life, whether that be after one or many
visits.

Contrary to many clinicians' fears, new medications for
treating severe mental illness will open new vistas for honing
and using psychotherapeutic skills and talents to make an
important impact on people's lives.

Appendix A

Prescribing Clozaril

In writing about psychotherapy for people recovering dramatically from years of mental illness we decided not to include a protocol for prescribing Clozaril in the body of the text. The focus was not on any particular medication, but on the psychotherapeutic treatment. Similarly, we did not include our observations of the risks and prevalence of side effects, drug-drug interactions, compliance, treatment of movement disorders, or the efficacy or titration of Clozaril with the dually diagnosed. However, we thought that this information might be of interest to some clinicians, including psychiatrists, psychiatric residents, and nurse clinical practitioners who have or are seeking prescribing privileges.

THE CLOZARIL CLINIC OF THE GREATER BRIDGEPORT COMMUNITY MENTAL HEALTH CENTER

We have the largest outpatient Clozaril program of the Department of Mental Health facilities in the State of Connecticut. Clozaril became available for general prescription use in 1991. Later that year, Title 19 (Medicaid) agreed to reimburse the cost of Clozaril, thereby resolving a thorny problem of who was to pay the estimated cost of $9,000 to $11,000 per year per patient. The Department of Mental Health required that each state facility set up clear written guidelines before admitting patients to a Clozaril program. The purpose of the requirement was twofold. The first was to ensure that every patient who was offered a trial of Clozaril met the inclusion criteria and would not be exposed to excessive risks. The second was to track people in the state mental health system taking Clozaril in a unique research study. In this section, we detail only the clinical aspects of the patient's care.

Eligibility

To be eligible for Clozaril a patient has to be over 18 years old, have a diagnosis of schizophrenia, have been afforded an unsatisfactory or incomplete remission from traditional neuroleptics, and/or have developed unacceptable side effects from those medications. Thus Clozaril, unlike Risperdal (risperidone), is not first-line treatment for schizophrenia. With growing evidence that Clozaril is helpful to patients with two other conditions, neuroleptic-dependent bipolar disorder and tardive dyskinesia, Clozaril can be offered to people with treatment-refractory illness. Additionally, the person must be free of myeloproliferative disease (illnesses affecting the bone marrow, causing increased white blood cell counts, such as leukemia) and not taking any other medication with the potential to suppress bone marrow function (the bone marrow makes blood cells). The patient has to be told that the medicine has the potential for suppressing the bone marrow and that his or her Social Security number and initials will be registered with the Clozaril National Registry. The patient must be willing to have blood drawn weekly for a white blood cell count. An information circular is reviewed with each patient and a copy given to each one (Appendix D). As Clozaril is approved by the Food and Drug Administration (FDA) for general prescription use, signed consent is not required. A rechallenge number must be issued that reflects that the patient has never had agranulocytosis or severe leukopenia caused by Clozaril and permits follow-up of the mandatory blood monitoring system. The Patient Safety Assurance Form (Form C) that contains all the information necessary for getting a rechallenge number appears at the end of this section. Additionally, the patient must have Title 19 or another means of paying for Clozaril.

Our eligibility requirements and the information circular about Clozaril for patients are found in Appendices B and D.

Titration

Although patients can start Clozaril during an inpatient admission, in our facility they most often begin taking Clozaril as outpatients. The patients therefore receive medicine according to the outpatient department's usual titration schedule. To ensure ease of compliance and to minimize dose-related discomfort or risks, the patient initiates Clozaril at 12.5 mg once or twice a day. Dosage increases are usually made every seven days by 25 mg once or twice a day as tolerated until a therapeutic dose is reached. This protocol is much slower than that recommended by Sandoz Pharmaceuticals. The patients therefore undergo an extended titration. Most people require a maintenance dose of 350 to 600 mg/day. People who have been psychotic for many years with extensive neuroleptic exposure histories may require a higher dose. The patients usually continue to take their pre-Clozaril medication, which is tapered as the Clozaril begins to show beneficial effects. The conventional antipsychotic (e.g., Haldol, Thorazine, or Prolixin) and antiparkinsonian medication (e.g.,

Cogentin or Artane) are usually the first medications to be tapered. Although most patients do very well while taking Clozaril alone, some (about 40 percent) require co-prescription of some other drug such as lithium carbonate or an antidepressant to maintain optimal symptom relief.

The therapeutic dose of Clozaril (i.e., the most effective amount) is usually reached in about three months. By that time, most or all of the prior medication has been discontinued.

The Most Common Side Effects

In clinical practice, drooling, sedation, weight gain, and constipation are the most commonly observed side effects. They can usually be relieved by such practical measures as placing a towel between the pillowcase and pillow, dose manipulation (taking divided doses, with the majority given before bedtime), calorie restriction, exercise, diet change, and stool softeners. The first three side effects (drooling, sedation, weight gain) typically disappear within six to twelve months of initiating treatment.

The Most Feared Side Effect

The most feared side effect is agranulocytosis. Agranulocytosis, or lack of granulocyte production due to the bone-marrow-suppressant effects of Clozaril, occurs in about 1 to 2 percent of people and is potentially fatal. Granulocytes account for more than half of the white blood cells. They are necessary for a person's immune system to function properly. The effect of bone marrow suppression is not dose related, although most reported cases occur during the first twenty weeks of treatment. There is no way of telling who will develop this effect.

The Clozaril National Registry provides a safety net for

people taking Clozaril. The Registry tracks the values of the weekly white blood cell count and withholds a rechallenge number if a person previously exposed to Clozaril has developed agranulocytosis. To assist the clinician in distinguishing agranulocytosis from leukopenia and reduced white blood cell count, we have included our clinical management protocol (Appendix B) for the differential diagnosis and treatment of each condition.

Seizures

Information provided by Sandoz stated that the incidence of seizures was higher than anticipated with conventional neuroleptics. The risk increases with doses over 600 mg/day.

Although we have many patients who take more than 600 mg of Clozaril a day, we have not seen any seizures attributable to the medication. A reasonable explanation of why seizures do not occur may lie in our slow titration, which probably reduces the chance of seizures. For the above reasons we do not automatically co-prescribe antiseizure medication for the prevention of convulsions.

Movement Disorders

Clozaril does not seem to cause tardive dystonia or tardive dyskinesia. Reports of cases of other extrapyramidal symptoms (parkinsonism) occurring while a person is taking clozapine are rare and not clearly causally linked to clozapine. We have not seen any new cases of tardive dyskinesia, tardive dystonia, or parkinsonism while a person has been taking Clozaril at our facility.

Moreover, many patients with moderate to severe tardive dyskinesia or dystonia have appreciated the reduction or elimination of these symptoms while taking Clozaril. Similarly, patients with treatment-resistant parkinsonian symptoms have benefited from the extinction of these disfiguring and sometimes also disabling symptoms. The improvement usually occurs within the first three months of treatment. The dose range of clozapine varies from 200 to 900 mg a day for patients with a pre-existing history of psychosis.

Dual Diagnosis

Like other inner-city community mental health centers, we treat many people with co-morbid severe schizophrenia and substance dependence or abuse. They are difficult to treat, are noncompliant with conventional treatment, and often have complex symptoms that defy accurate diagnosis, especially while they are abusing. Such people comprise more than half of our patient census.

When dually diagnosed patients become abstinent, we notice that they actually suffer from a variety of conditions. In fact, the term *dual-diagnosis* is a misnomer for the many who suffer from more than two conditions. Furthermore, a significant number of dually diagnosed people tell us that they use illegal drugs and/or alcohol in order to feel normal, rather than to get high. At least some of them do not feel normal because they suffer from painful or dysphoric symptoms of residual schizophrenia or from negative symptoms induced by conventional neuroleptics. For these people, taking drugs is a desperate attempt to self-medicate unbearable symptoms. It stands to reason that when they obtain better symptom relief from prescribed medication, they stop abusing drugs, sometimes without significant involvement in recovery programs.

Given the above observations, it is not surprising that any medication that gives better symptom relief to the self-medicators will be better accepted and has the potential to alleviate illegal drug use. We are not alone in noticing the efficacy of Clozaril for the dually diagnosed. Buckley and colleagues (1994a,b) have formally studied such patients. The patients do very well, often entering a significant and astonishing recovery from both schizophrenia and substance dependence or abuse.

There are some real difficulties in offering Clozaril to the dually diagnosed who are outpatients, actively abusing, and have histories of noncompliance with treatment. In our experience, to maximize patient safety and cooperation two treatment tools must almost always be utilized. First, patients must accept a voluntary money management program in which the facility or designee is a co-payee of their benefit checks (entitlements). Patients often make the commitment to this program not based on true insight but because they see the money management program as giving them an express ticket out of the hospital, a pack of cigarettes, and a few dollars in their pocket every day. After discharge from the inpatient unit, they come to the center daily for a twofold purpose: to get their medicine (staff monitored) and then their cigarettes and money. The weekly blood draw is combined with the medication supervision before entitlements are distributed. The second critical ingredient is a slow titration of Clozaril, with frequent follow-up visits and a goal of finding a minimum effective dose. The dictum, "go slow, stay low" (also seen as "start low, go slow"), is the same policy we would use in medicating the medically ill or geriatric patient. After three months, most patients are ready to resume a higher level of independent function and have suspended their illegal drug use. Return of the autonomy to manage their own money and take their medicine is frequently established within two years for most patients.

CLOZARIL®
(clozapine)
Patient Safety Assurance Form

SUBMIT TO: CLOZARIL National Registry   OR   PHONE: 1-800-448-5938
              Sandoz Pharmaceuticals Corporation
              59 Route 10
              East Hanover, NJ 07936

Patient Initials: ☐ ☐   Date of Birth*: ☐ ☐ ☐   Patient Social Security #: ☐ ☐ ☐ ☐ ☐ ☐
                  First Last   M D Y

Sex: ☐ ☐   Patient Zip Code: ☐ ☐ ☐ ☐
     M F

Today's Date: ☐ ☐ ☐   RACE: ☐ ☐ ☐ ☐ ☐
              M D Y   W B Hisp Oriental Other

Patient New to CLOZARIL (clozapine): ☐   Patient Continuing on CLOZARIL: ☐

RECHALLENGE CLEARANCE AUTHORIZATION NUMBER ☐ ☐ - ☐ ☐ ☐ ☐ ☐
(Assigned by the CLOZARIL National Registry)

1. I am completely familiar with CLOZARIL package labeling, including WARNINGS concerning the risk of death associated with agranulocytosis.

2. To limit "rechallenge" of patients at risk, I understand that each patient must be enrolled in the CLOZARIL National Registry. Since CLOZARIL (clozapine) should not be prescribed prior to receiving a patient-specific rechallenge clearance authorization number from the National Registry, I agree to promptly report all WBC counts/evaluations (normal and abnormal) to the pharmacy for submission to the CLOZARIL National Registry within 7 days of collection. I also agree to notify the CLOZARIL National Registry promptly of all discontinued patients, and submit to the National Registry the results of the four required weekly blood tests after discontinuation of therapy.

3. I understand that the CLOZARIL Safety Support Team will work with local Quality Assurance Committees to help ensure adherence to CLOZARIL package insert requirements. Sandoz will not make on-site audits and will not be privy to patients' names.

Physician's Signature _____   ☐ ☐ ☐   Physician's DEA/ID Number ☐ ☐ ☐ ☐ ☐ ☐
                                                M D Y

Physician's Name (typed or printed) & Title _____   Address _____

Physician's Phone Number _____   City, State _____   Physician's Zip Code ☐ ☐ ☐ ☐ ☐

*Safety and efficacy in children under 16 has not been established.

This is a three-part, NCR (no carbon required) form. First copy (white) is sent to the CLOZARIL National Registry, Sandoz Pharmaceuticals Corporation, 59 Route 10, East Hanover, NJ 07936. Second copy (blue) becomes part of the pharmacist's record. Third copy (yellow) remains with the prescribing physician. The Rechallenge Clearance Authorization Number must appear on the pharmacy copy prior to initial dispensing.

© 1991 Sandoz Pharmaceuticals Corporation   Printed in U.S.A.   CLO-4013   3/91

Appendix B

Greater Bridgeport Community Mental Health Center Clozapine Protocol

I. INCLUSION CRITERIA: (All answers must be "yes" or clozapine cannot be prescribed)

Yes   No

____   ____ 1. Patient is at least 18 years old.

____   ____ 2. Diagnosis of schizophrenia or schizoaffective disorder.

____   ____ 3. At least two adequate trials on different antipsychotic medications (e.g., either a dose equivalent to 1,000 mg of chlorpromazine per day for six weeks or the production of unacceptable side effects; at least one of the drug trials must have been a nonphenothiazine), or

____   ____ 4. Lack of a history of adequate symptom relief without unacceptable side effects on any antipsychotic medication other than clozapine.

Yes   No

___   ___   5. Absence of a current myeloproliferative disorder.

___   ___   6. Absence of clozapine-induced severe leukopenia.

___   ___   7. Absence of a current WBC count of less than
3,500.

___   ___   8. Absence of a current granulocyte count below
1,500.

___   ___   9. Absence of current CNS depression.

___   ___   10. Absence of current debilitated physical state.

___   ___   11. Absence of pregnancy or production of breast
milk.

___   ___   12. Absence of concurrent use of drugs that may
suppress bone marrow function.

___   ___   13. Patient has a source of payment or Medicaid
application has been submitted.

II. PROCEDURE FOR PRESCRIBING CLOZAPINE:

1. The risks and benefits of clozapine (including the need for
weekly blood drawing, the risk of agranulocytosis, and the
fact that the patient's Social Security number and initials
will be entered into the Sandoz National Registry (Sandoz
Pharmaceuticals Corporation, 59 Route 10, East Hanover,
NJ, 07936) will be discussed with the patient and that

discussion will be documented in the patient's chart. The patient will be given a copy of *Information About Clozapine* (Appendix D).

2. Spanish-speaking patients will receive explanations in their own language and literature to read in Spanish (when available).

3. When indicated, the patient will sign a standard GBCMHC release form to permit discussion with a physician who may be prescribing nonpsychiatric medication(s).

4. Form A (Patient Safety Understandings Form), signed by the Medical Director and the participating pharmacist, has been submitted to Sandoz. The Center is enrolled in the "Treatment System."

5. Form C (Patient Safety Assurance Form) will be completed and a rechallenge number will be assigned to each patient. A copy of form C will be kept in the chart.

6. Form D or E (National Registry WBC Count Reporting Form) will be completed weekly for each patient. One copy will be kept in the medical record, and two copies will be sent to the pharmacy. The pharmacy will keep one copy and then submit the other to the National Registry at Sandoz on a weekly basis.

7. A baseline medical evaluation will be completed, and will include the following:

   a. Chemistry screening panel
   b. CBC
   c. Pregnancy test (only when indicated)

8. The general procedure for prescribing clozapine (after steps 1–7 have been completed) will be the following:

a. The patients will meet with a physician and nurse at a weekly clozapine clinic every Wednesday morning. One half-hour prior to this visit, the patient will have his/her blood drawn at the Center by a Metpath technician. The blood will be transported by the technician back to Metpath for analysis.

NOTE: Laboratory reports are generally available within two days and are printed out on Metpath computer forms here at the Center. Laboratory results will also be sent directly to Alliance Pharmacy by the nurse coordinator at GBCMHC.

b. Each patient on clozapine will have a specially marked chart. The clozapine nurse coordinator will be certain each chart is present the evening before the next scheduled visit and that the most recent WBC count (one that has been drawn within one week of the current visit) is affixed to the chart if it has not already been reviewed.

In the event the WBC report is unavailable, the nurse coordinator will obtain the WBC result from the computer located on the sixth floor, after having notified Metpath about the need for the WBC result. She will then affix the WBC report to the chart. The psychiatrist will review the results of the WBC and, using the guidelines from the *Clinical Management of Reduced White Blood Cell Count, Leukopenia, and Agranulocytosis* (Appendix C), will determine if the prescription can be written.

No clozapine prescription can be written unless the patient has a blood level drawn, and the psy-

chiatrist determines that the results of the past week's WBC count are acceptable.

c. If the criteria listed above are met, a prescription for clozapine (written for one week only), will be FAXed to the contract pharmacy, Reliance Health Services. After reviewing the results of the WBC and having found them acceptable, the pharmacy will fill the prescription and deliver it to GBCMHC. The pharmacy will then submit the WBC reporting form to Sandoz.

d. The dose of clozapine will be increased according to the guidelines established by Sandoz, increasing as rapidly as is safely possible. In accordance with those guidelines, the maximum dose that can be administered at one time is 450 mg. Doses above 450 mg must be divided and given twice a day. The maximum daily dose is 900 mg.

e. The Brief Psychiatric Rating Scale (BPRS) will be administered prior to the initiation of treatment, at three and six months of treatment, and yearly thereafter.

III. PROCEDURE FOR DISCONTINUING CLOZAPINE:

1. Clozapine will be discontinued for any of the three following reasons:

   a. The patient refuses to have the weekly WBC drawn, and cannot be persuaded otherwise, or

   b. The patient develops unacceptable side effects, including, but not limited to, clinically significant agranulocytosis, or

   c. The patient has been given an adequate clinical trial of clozapine (within a six-month period), but has not shown a significant positive response to warrant continuation of the medication.

An adequate trial is that which represents the maximum allowable dose, the maximum dose tolerated by the patient, or the dose on which the patient responds sufficiently to be discharged from the hospital.

A significant positive response is defined as a 30 percent decrease in the Brief Psychiatric Rating Scale (BPRS) score.

If either the patient or the treating psychiatrist believes that the patient has responded significantly to clozapine, even though the BPRS score has not dropped 30 percent, an appeal can be initiated by either the patient or the psychiatrist to the Chief of Professional Services, whose decision will be final. Documentation of the content and findings of such appeals will be sent to the Office of the Commissioner (OOC) within one week of the appeal hearing. (The patient will be continued on clozapine during the appeal process unless this is medically contraindicated).

Once the decision to stop clozapine has been made, clozapine will be tapered and discontinued as rapidly as can be done safely.

2. If clozapine is discontinued, a WBC will be drawn weekly on Wednesday morning for four weeks. If an appointment is missed, outreach will be done (e.g., clinical staff from the Center will call the patient and ask them to come in for blood testing. If they refuse or cannot be reached by phone, Center staff will go to their places of residence and, if they agree, bring them either to the Center for blood testing or take them directly to Columbia Medical Laboratory. If

necessary, a certified letter will be sent to the patients informing them of the necessity of having their blood drawn.

IV. ANTICIPATED PROBLEMS AND THEIR SOLUTIONS:

1. Patient misses appointment:

   If an appointment is missed, outreach will be done. Clinical staff from the Center will call patients and ask them to come in for blood testing. If they refuse or cannot be reached by phone, Center staff will go to their place of residence and, if they agree, bring them either to the Center for blood testing or take them directly to Columbia Medical Laboratory. If necessary, a certified letter will be sent to the patients informing them of the need for blood testing.

2. Patient refuses WBC:

   Find the means to persuade the patient of the importance of cooperating. Enlist the support of family members in this process. If the patient continues to refuse WBC testing, the patient will not be given any further clozapine and will be dropped from the program. At a minimum, however, further attempts will be made to obtain WBC testing for four weeks after the last dose of clozapine (see "1" above).

   Note: Clinical staff includes nurses, social workers, and mental health workers.

3. Patient's WBC count drops below 3,500 or the granulocyte count drops below 1,500:

   See the Clinical Management Protocol.

4. Patient's clozapine is lost or stolen:

   A small supply of clozapine will be kept in the GBCMHC pharmacy and MOD pharmacy that can be dispensed at any time such a need arises (twenty-four hours/day, seven days/week).

5. The patient is found to lack two adequate trials on different antipsychotic medications.

   Clozapine will be tapered and discontinued in a medically appropriate and timely fashion, after discussing the need to do so with the patient. Adequate antipsychotic medication trials, as defined above (see Inclusion Criteria, part I-3), will be started.

Appendix C

Greater Bridgeport Community Mental Health Center Clinical Management of Reduced White Blood Cell Count, Leukopenia, and Agranulocytosis

PROBLEM	Reduced White Blood Cell Count
WBC FINDINGS	WBC count reveals a significant drop (even if WBC count is still in normal range). Significant drop =
	1. drop of over 3,000 cells from prior tests, or
	2. three or more consecutive drops in WBC counts
CLINICAL FINDINGS	Patients show no symptoms of infection.
TREATMENT	1. Monitor patient closely.
	2. Institute twice-weekly CBC

tests with differentials, if deemed appropriate by attending physician

3. Clozaril may continue.

PROBLEM   Mild leukopenia

WBC FINDINGS   WBC = 3,000–3,500

CLINICAL FINDINGS   Patient may or may not show clinical symptoms such as lethargy, fever, sore throat, weakness.

TREATMENT   1. Monitor patient closely.

                        2. Institute a minimum of twice-weekly CBC tests with differentials.

                        3. Clozaril may continue.

PROBLEM   Leukopenia or Granulocytopenia

WBC FINDINGS   WBC = 2,000–3,000 or granulocytes = 1,000–1,500.

CLINICAL FINDINGS   Patient may or may not show clinical symptoms such as fever, sore throat, lethargy, weakness.

TREATMENT   1. Interrupt Clozaril at once.

                        2. Institute Daily CBC tests with differentials.

3. Increase medical supervision and consult a hematologist.

4. Clozaril may be resumed after normalization of WBC.

PROBLEM	Agranulocytosis (uncomplicated)
WBC FINDINGS	WBC below 2,000 or granulocytes below 1,000.
CLINICAL FINDINGS	None.
TREATMENT	

1. Discontinue Clozaril at once.

2. Transfer patient to a general hospital or, if an outpatient, bring to an emergency department with a copy of the WBC.

3. The patient may be placed in protective isolation.

4. Obtain a hematology consultation and consider bone marrow biopsy to determine if progenitor cells are being suppressed.

5. Do a WBC count every two days until count returns to normal (about 2–3 weeks).

6. Avoid use of medication with bone-marrow-suppressing potential; Clozaril cannot be restarted.

7. Consider use of antibiotics.

PROBLEM   Agranulocytosis (with complica-
                        tions)

WBC FINDINGS   WBC below 2,000 or granulo-
                        cytes below 1,000.

CLINICAL FINDINGS   Patient shows definite evidence
                        of infection such as fever, sore
                        throat, lethargy, weakness, mal-
                        aise, skin ulcerations, rash, etc.

TREATMENT   Follow 1 to 7 above plus

8. Obtain a hematology or
    infectious disease consulta-
    tion to determine appro-
    priate antibiotic regimen.

9. Clozaril cannot be
    prescribed.

10. Psychiatrist must prescribe
    appropriate medication
    (usually lorazapem or halo-
    peridol) if needed for con-
    trol of psychotic symptoms
    to ensure patient comfort
    and capacity to cooperate
    with medical treatment.

PROBLEM   Recovery from Agranulocytosis

WBC FINDINGS   WBC over 4,000 and granulo-
                        cytes over 2,000.

CLINICAL FINDINGS   Patient shows no symptoms of
                     infection.

TREATMENT   1. Institute once-weekly CBC
                        test with differential for four
                        consecutive normal values.

                     2. Clozaril *must not* be restarted.

Appendix D

Greater Bridgeport Community Mental Health Center Information about Clozapine

WHAT IS CLOZAPINE?

Clozapine is a medicine that has been found to help *some* people with schizophrenia or similar conditions, even though standard medications they have taken haven't worked very well or have caused unacceptable side effects.

Clozapine became available in the United States in 1991, although it has been used in Europe for a number of years. The brand name for clozapine is Clozaril.

WHY AM I BEING OFFERED CLOZAPINE?

You are being offered clozapine because your medical records show that you have not completely responded to at least two standard medications for your psychiatric illness in the past, or side effects from your medications have been too severe.

The standard medications that are available to treat

schizophrenia and related conditions include: Thorazine (chlorpromazine), Mellaril (thioridazine), Haldol (haloperidol), Prolixin (fluphenazine), Navane (thiothixene), Stelazine (trifluoperazine), Trilafon (perphenazine), Moban (molindone), and Loxitane (loxapin).

If you are currently on a standard medication, you may be experiencing side effects from them now, like dizziness, dry mouth, stiffness, restlessness, blurred vision, constipation, or other side effects.

The standard medications may also cause long-term side effects, the most common being tardive dyskinesia or TD. TD means abnormal movements of the lips, toes, tongue, jaw, arms or legs, and body that sometimes continue even after the medicine is stopped.

In addition, these standard medications do not work for everyone.

WHAT BENEFITS CAN I EXPECT IF I TAKE CLOZAPINE?

Clozapine offers the hope that your condition will improve to a greater extent than it has with standard medications and with fewer side effects.

Clozapine *may* have fewer undesirable side effects. Clozapine is less likely to cause stiffness or restlessness often caused by other medications. Clozapine is also less likely to cause abnormal involuntary movements such as tardive dyskinesia or TD. In fact, if you already have abnormal movements, it is possible that clozapine will help control or eliminate these movements.

WHAT ARE THE POSSIBLE PROBLEMS CAUSED BY TAKING CLOZAPINE?

For some people, clozapine has undesirable side effects that are different from the side effects of the medicines you have been taking.

Relatively Common Side Effects

1. sleepiness
2. excess saliva
3. fast heart rate
4. dizziness
5. constipation
6. weight gain

Less Common Side Effects

1. low blood pressure (especially in the beginning of treatment)
2. headache
3. tremor
4. fainting
5. sweating
6. dry mouth
7. nausea
8. visual problems

Rare but Serious Side Effects

About one person in fifty who takes clozapine will have a decrease of the white blood cells. This can lead to a life-threatening infection, but most people recover completely with proper medical treatment.

The early warning signs of this reaction, called "agranulocytosis," include feeling tired, having a fever or a sore throat, or getting sores that do not heal. (If you decide to take clozapine and have these problems, it is important to report them to your doctor immediately.)

If you decide to take clozapine, your doctor will monitor your white cell count by obtaining weekly blood counts. This means that each week a needle will be stuck in one of your

veins and a small amount of blood will be drawn. This procedure may cause discomfort and bruising.

The company that makes clozapine (Sandoz) *requires* that
the doctor prescribing clozapine for a patient send that patient's initials (but not the full name), Social Security number
or substitute number, and the results of that patient's blood
tests to a National Data Bank. This is so that a person who has
a bad reaction to clozapine will not be given clozapine again
and so that the drug's maker can watch for signs that a person's
white blood count is getting too low.

Thus, your blood will have to be tested once a week with
the results of this test going to the company that makes
clozapine for as long as you continue to take this medication.

WHAT ELSE DO I NEED TO KNOW ABOUT IF I TAKE CLOZAPINE?

Pregnancy:
> You should tell your doctor if you become pregnant,
> plan to get pregnant, or are breast feeding, since cloza-
> pine may not be safe in these conditions.

Driving and other hazardous activity:
> These activities should be avoided while starting cloza-
> pine.

Drinking or taking over-the-counter medicines:
> Drinking should be avoided. Discuss over-the-counter
> medicines with your doctor before taking them. Also
> discuss any other medicines you are taking with your
> doctor. Do not take Tegretol.

WHAT HAPPENS IF I TAKE CLOZAPINE BUT THEN I WANT TO STOP?

If you take clozapine but later decide to stop, we cannot
promise that you will be able to restart it if you want to. You

will continue to be able to have the other standard medications, however.

WHAT HAPPENS IF I DON'T GET BETTER ON CLOZAPINE?

If you take clozapine and it turns out not to benefit you more than your usual medications, you will have been exposed to clozapine's side effects without any benefit. Therefore, if you try clozapine for six months and it does not help you significantly, you will be taken off clozapine and offered other standard treatments.

WHAT DO I DO IF I HAVE QUESTIONS ABOUT CLOZAPINE?

Please feel free to discuss clozapine with your doctor any time you have questions. Other staff members will also be able to answer many of your questions.

References

Alanen, Y. O. (1966). The family in the pathogenesis of schizophrenia and neurotic disorders. *Acta Psychiatrica Scandinavica* 42, Suppl. 189.

Allport, G. W. (1982). *The Nature of Prejudice*. Reading, MA: Addison-Wesley Publishing Company.

Andreasen, N. C., Arndt, S., Alliger, R., et al. (1995). Symptoms of schizophrenia. *Archives of General Psychiatry* 52:341–351.

Beck, J. C., and van der Kolk, B. A. (1987). Reports of childhood incest and current behavior of chronically hospitalized psychotic women. *American Journal of Psychiatry* 144:1474–1476.

Bordman, G. M. (1978). *American Musical Theatre: A Chronicle*. New York: Oxford University Press.

Buckley, P., Thompson, P., Way, L., and Meltzer, H. Y. (1994a). Substance abuse among patients with treatment-resistant schizophrenia: characteristics and implications for clozapine therapy. *American Journal of Psychiatry* 151:385–389.

————— (1994b). Substance abuse and clozapine treatment. *Journal of Clinical Psychiatry* 55:114–116.

Bulfinch, T. (1942). *The Age of Fable*. New York: Heritage.

Carmen, E. (H.), Rieker, P. P., and Mills, T. (1984). Victims of violence and psychiatric illness. *American Journal of Psychiatry* 141:378–383.

Carpenter, W. T., Strauss, J. S., and Muleh, S. (1973). Are there pathogno-monic symptoms in schizophrenia? *Archives of General Psychiatry* 28:847–850.

Casey, D. E., and Hansen, T. E. (1984). Spontaneous dyskinesias. In *Neuropsychiatric Movement Disorders,* ed. D. V. Jeste and R. J. Wyatt, pp. 67–96. Washington, DC: American Psychiatric Press.

Chiu, H. F., Lam, L. C., Chan, C. H., et al. (1987). Clinical and polygraphic characteristics of patients with respiratory dyskinesia. *British Journal of Psychiatry* 162:828–830.

Corrigan, P. W., Yudofsky, S. C., and Silver, J. M. (1993). Pharmacological and behavioral treatments for aggressive psychiatric inpatients. *Hospital and Community Psychiatry* 44:125–133.

Cournos, F., McKinnon, K., Meyer-Bahlburg, H., et al. (1993). HIV risk activity among persons with severe mental illness: preliminary findings. *Hospital and Community Psychiatry* 44:1104–1106.

Courtois, C. (1988). *Healing the Incest Wound.* New York: Norton.

Craine, I. S., Henson, C. E., Colliver, J. A., et al. (1988). Prevalence of a history of sexual abuse among female psychiatric patients in a state hospital system. *Hospital and Community Psychiatry* 39:300–304.

Degen, K. (1982). Sexual dysfunction in women using major tranquilizers. *Psychosomatics* 23:959–961.

Degen, K., Cole, N., Tamayo, L., and Dzerovych, G. (1990). Intensive case management for the seriously mentally ill. *Administration and Policy in Mental Health* 17:265–269.

den Herder, D., and Redner, L. (1991). The treatment of childhood sexual trauma in chronically mentally ill adults. *Health and Social Work* 16(1):50–57.

Dewald, P. A. (1994). Principles of supportive psychotherapy. *American Journal of Psychotherapy* 48:4, 505–518.

Diagnostic and Statistical Manual of Mental Disorders. (1994). 4th ed. Washington, DC: American Psychiatric Association.

Eichelman, B. (1987). Neurochemical and psychopharmacologic aspects of aggressive behavior. In *Psychopharmacology: The Third Generation of Progress,* ed. H. Y. Meltzer, pp. 697–704. New York: Raven.

Ellason, J. W., and Ross, C. A. (1995). Positive and negative symptoms in dissociative identity disorder and schizophrenia: a comparative analysis. *Journal of Nervous and Mental Disease* 183(4):236–241.

Ellenberger, H. F. (1970). *The Discovery of the Unconscious.* New York: Basic

Books.

Fenton, W. S. (1995). Negative symptoms in schizophrenia. *Clinical Advances in the Treatment of Psychiatric Disorder* 9(l):16, 13–14.

Fenton, W. S., Wyatt, R. J., and McGlashan, T. H. (1994). Risk factors for spontaneous dyskinesia in schizophrenia. *Archives of General Psychiatry* 51:643–649.

Fink, D., and Golinkoff, M. (1990). MPD, borderline personality disorder, and schizophrenia: a comparative study of clinical features. *Dissociation* 3:127–134.

Ghadirian A. M., Lehmann, H. E., Dongier, M., and Kolivakis, T. (1985). Multiple personality in a case of functional psychosis. *Comprehensive Psychiatry* 26(l):22–28.

Glazer, W. M., Morgenstern, H., and Doucette, J. T. (1993). Predicting the long-term risk of tardive dyskinesia in outpatients maintained on neuroleptic medications. *Journal of Clinical Psychiatry* 54:133–139.

Goffman, E. (1961). *Asylums.* New York: Doubleday.

Herman, J. L. (1991). *Trauma and Recovery.* New York: Basic Books.

Jacobson, A. (1989). Physical and sexual assault histories among psychiatric outpatients. *American Journal of Psychiatry* 146:755–758.

Janssen, P. A., Niemegeers, J. E., Anwouters, F., et al. (1987). Pharmacology of risperidone, a new antipsychotic with serotonin-S2 and dopamine-D2 antagonistic properties. *The Journal of Pharmacology and Experimental Therapeutics* 244:685–693.

Kates, J., and Rockland, L. H. (1994). Supportive psychotherapy of the schizophrenic patient. *American Journal of Psychotherapy* 48(4):543–561.

Kay, S. R., Fiszbein, A., and Opler, L. A. (1987). The positive and negative syndrome scale (PANSS) for schizophrenia. *Schizophrenia Bulletin* 13(2):261–276.

Kesselring, J. (1941). *Arsenic and Old Lace.* New York: Random House.

Kestenbaum, K. (1993). *Adolescent psychotherapy.* Paper presented at the symposia of the New England Educational Institute, Eastham, MA, August.

Kipling, R. (1894). *The Jungle Book.* London: Macmillan.

Kluft, R. P. (1985). *Childhood Antecedents of Multiple Personality.* Washington, DC: American Psychiatric Press.

_____ (1987). First rank symptoms as diagnostic indicators to multiple personality disorder. *American Journal of Psychiatry* 144:292–298.

_____ (1990). *Incest Related Syndromes of Adult Psychopathology*. Washington, DC: American Psychiatric Press.

Kraepelin, E. L. (1919). *Textbook of Psychiatry: Dementia Praecox.* London: McMillan.

Larson, L. R. (1995). Maxine Mason's last days. Letter to the Editor. *The New Yorker,* April 3, p. 10.

Lidz, T., Fleck, S., and Cornelison, A. (1965). *Schizophrenia and the Family.* New York: International Universities Press.

Lidz, T., and Lidz, R. W. (1982). The curative factors in psychotherapy of schizophrenic disorders. In *Curative Factors in Dynamic Psychiatry,* ed. S. Slipp, pp. 1–38. New York: McGraw-Hill.

Marder, S. R., and Meibach, R. C. (1994). Risperidone in the treatment of schizophrenia. *American Journal of Psychiatry* 151:825–841.

McGorry, P. D., Chanen A., McCarthy, E., et al. (1991). Posttraumatic stress disorder following recent-onset psychosis. *Journal of Nervous and Mental Disease* 179(5):253–258.

Meltzer, H. Y., Burnett, S., Bastani, B., and Ramirez, L. F. (1990). Effects of six months of clozapine treatment on the quality of life of chronic schizophrenic patients. *Hospital and Community Psychiatry* 41:892–897.

Muenzenmaier, K., Meyer, I., Struening, E., and Ferber, J. (1993). Childhood abuse and neglect among women outpatients with chronic mental illness. *Hospital and Community Psychiatry* 44(7):666–670.

Nasper, E., and Smith, T. (1995). Treatment of multiple personality disorder in a community mental health center. In *Dissociative Identity Disorder,* ed. L. Cohen, J. Berzoff, and M. Elin, pp. 493–507. Northvale, NJ: Jason Aronson.

Quimby, L. G., Andrei, A., and Putnam, F. W. (1993). The deinstitutionalization of patients with chronic multiple personality disorder. In *Clinical Perspectives on Multiple Personality Disorder,* ed. R. P. Kluft and C. G. Fine, pp. 201–225. Washington, DC: American Psychiatric Press.

Rose, S. M., Peabody, C. G. and Stratigeas, B. (1991). Undetected abuse among intensive case management clients. *Hospital and Community Psychiatry* 42(6):499–503.

Ross, C. A. (1989). *Multiple Personality Disorder: Diagnosis, Clinical Features and Treatment.* New York: Wiley.

Ross, C. A., Anderson, G., and Clark, P. (1994). Childhood abuse and the positive symptoms of schizophrenia. *Hospital and Community Psychiatry* 45(5):489–491.

Ross, C. A., Miller, S. D., Reagor, P., et al. (1990). Schneiderian symptoms in multiple personality disorder and schizophrenia. *Comprehensive Psychiatry* 31:111–118.

Ross, C. A., and Norton, G. R. (1988). Multiple personality disorder patients with a prior diagnosis of schizophrenia. *Dissociation* 1(2):39–42.

Sacks, O. (1974). *Awakenings*. New York: Doubleday.

Spaniol, L. (1995). Recovery from serious mental illness: a review of the research and implications for supporting recovery. Paper presented at the Janssen Pharmaceutica CNS Roundtable, Boston, MA, June.

Stern, D. (1985). *The Interpersonal World of the Infant*. New York: Basic Books.

Strauss, J .S. (1989). Subjective experiences in schizophrenia: toward a new dynamic psychiatry—II. *Schizophrenia Bulletin* 15(2):179–187.

Tardiff, K. (1992). The current state of psychiatry in the treatment of violent patients. *Archives of General Psychiatry* 49:493–499.

Turner, T. (1989). Rich and mad in Victorian England. *Psychological Medicine* 19:29–44.

van der Kolk, B. A. (1987). *Psychological Trauma*. Washington, DC: American Psychiatric Press.

van der Kolk, B. A., and van der Hart, O. (1989). Pierre Janet and the breakdown of adaptation in psychological trauma. *American Journal of Psychiatry* 146(12):1530–1540.

Wagner, J. (1986). *The Search for Signs of Intelligent Life in the Universe*. New York: Harper & Row.

Webster's Encyclopedic Unabridged Dictionary of the English Language (1989). New York: Gramercy Books.

Winnicott, D. W. (1960). The theory of the parent–infant relationship. *International Journal of Psycho-Analysis* 41:585–595.

Yassa, R., Nair, N. P., Iskandar, H., and Schwartz, G. (1990). Factors in the development of severe forms of tardive dyskinesia. *American Journal of Psychiatry* 147:1156–1163.

Yudofsky, S. C., Silver, J. M., Jackson, W., et al. (1986). The overt aggression scale for the objective rating of verbal and physical aggression. *American Journal of Psychiatry* 143:35–39.

Credits

The authors gratefully acknowledge permission to reprint material from the following sources:

Arsenic and Old Lace, by Joseph Kesselring. Copyright © 1941 by Random House, Inc.

The Marriage of Cadmus and Harmony, by Robert Colasso. Copyright © 1993 by Alfred A. Knopf.

The Search for Signs of Intelligent Life in the Universe, by Jane Wagner. Copyright © 1986 by Jane Wagner Inc. Reprinted by permission of HarperCollins Publications, Inc. and Jane Wagner Inc.

"American Pie," words and music by Don McLean. Copyright © 1971, 1972 Music Corporation of America, a division of MCA, Inc., and Benny Bird Music. All rights controlled and administered by Music Corporation of America, a division of MCA, Inc. All rights reserved. International copyright secured. Used by permission.

Index

Abuse. *See* Sexual molestation
Adolescence, schizophrenia
    and, 93
Aggression. *See* Violence
Agranulocytosis, Clozaril, 6–7,
    82, 188, 198–199,
    215–219
Akathisia, described, 25–26
Alanen, Y. O., 93
Alcoholics Anonymous, 97
Alcoholism, schizophrenia and,
    96–97, 109–110
Allport, G. W., 120
Andreasen, N. C., 35
Annoyance, reacting with,
    negative and positive
    symptoms, 40
Antiparkinsonians, 24
Antipsychotics. *See* Clozaril
Assertive Community

Treatment Program, 79,
    80, 95
Avoidance, reacting with,
    negative and positive
    symptoms, 40

Baseline, meaning of, 184–186
Beck, J. C., 155
Bone marrow suppression,
    Clozaril, 6–7, 82, 188,
    198–199, 215–219
Bordman, G. M., 65
Bradykinesia, described, 26–27
Brain, imaging of, 184
Buckley, P., 109, 200
Bulfinch, T., 108, 179

Calasso, R., 107, 119, 163, 170
Carmen, E., 155
Carpenter, W. T., 153

Case management,
    deinstitutionalization and,
    75
Casey, D. E., 19
Cataplexy, dopamine blockade
    and, 22–23
Child abuse. *See* Sexual
    molestation
Clozaril
    delusion and, 151–152
    dual diagnosis and, 200–201
    effects and side effects, 6–8,
        82, 101, 198–200
    eligibility for, 196–197
    informational sheet on,
        223–227
    initial prescription of, 45–46
    introduction of, 5–6
    medication group, 166–168
    as mixed blessing, 9–13,
        46–51
    movement disorders and, 29
    protocol for, 205–212
    psychotherapy and, 117,
        143–145, 165
    racism and, 121
    reimbursement for, 196
    sexuality and, 114, 141
    substance abuse and,
        109–110
    titration, 197–198
    violence and, 112, 122–124,
        133–135
Corrigan, P., 111
Cournos, F., 113
Courtois, C., 155–156
Craine, I. S., 155
Culture
    mental illness and, 182–184

    nonrational thinking,
        181–182

Davis, W., 17, 33
Degen, K., 75, 113
Deinstitutionalization,
    psychotherapy and, 74–88
Delusion
    Clozaril and, 151–152
    good and evil in, 131
    schizophrenia and, 94–95
den Herder, D., 155
Dewald, P. A., 169
Dissociative personality
    disorder
    Clozaril and, 151–152
    schizophrenia and,
        differential diagnosis,
        152–157
    sexual molestation, 154–156
Dopamine, 9, 188
Dopamine blockade, cataplexy
    and, 22–23
Dyskinesia
    biology of, 21–23
    drug-induced, 20–21, 98
    spontaneous, 19–20
Dystonia, described, 25

Eichelman, B., 111
Eligibility, for Clozaril,
    196–197
Ellason, J. W., 154
Ellenberger, H. F., 153, 155

Family life
    improvement consequences
        and, 50
    schizophrenia and, 92

Feelings group. *See also*
    Psychotherapy
  case illustration, 101–103
  origins of, 52–53
  sanity, case histories of
      reaction to, 59–70,
      87–88
Feminism, 180
Fenton, W. S., 20, 35, 36
Fink, D., 154
Food and Drug Administration
    (FDA), 22
Freud, S., 155

Genital mutilation, 149
Ghadirian, A. M., 154
Glazer, W. M., 20
Goffman, E., 74
Golinkoff, M., 154
Good and evil, in delusion, 131
Grieving, as consequence of
    improvement, 47–48
Group psychotherapy. *See*
    Feelings group;
    Psychotherapy

Haldol, 12, 19
Hallucination
  negative and positive
      symptoms, 37–38
  schizophrenia and, 94–95
Hansen, T. E., 19
Herman, J. L., 51
Homosexuality, schizophrenia
    and, 115–116
Hope, meaning of, 186

Individuation, schizophrenia
    and, 93

Interpersonal relationships,
    ambivalence toward,
    83–85
Irrationality. *See* Nonrational
    thinking
Irving, W., 5

Jacobson, A., 155
Janssen, P. A., 8

Kay, S. R., 153
Kesselring, J., xi, 59
Kestenbaum, C., 93
Kipling, R., 129, 130, 131, 145
Kluft, R. P., 153, 155, 156
Kraepelin, E. L., 19

Larson, L. R., 45, 48
Lerner, A. J., 65
Lidz, R. W., 53, 93
Lidz, T., 53, 93
Loss, improvement
    consequences and, 50

Magnetic resonance imaging,
    mental illness and, 184
Marder, S. R., 8
Masturbation. *See* Sexuality
McGorry, P. D., 51
McLean, D., 91, 100
Medication group, described,
    166–168
Meilbach, R. C., 8
Meltzer, H. Y., 7
Mental illness. *See*
    Schizophrenia
Movement disorders. *See also*
    Dyskinesia
  Clozaril and, 199–200

Movement disorders. *(continued)*
descriptive categorization of, 23–27
Muenzenmaier, K., 155
Myoclonic movement, described, 26

Nasper, E., 156
Negative symptoms
defined, 35–37
impact of, on clinician, 37–41
Neglect, reacting with, negative and positive symptoms, 40–41
Neurotransmitters, schizophrenia and, 187–190
Nonrational thinking, relevance of, 181–182
Norms, group therapy and, 170–171
Norton, G. R., 154

Olanzapine, 8
described, 189

Parkinsonian tremor
Clozaril and, 199–200
described, 26
Parkinson's disease, 9
Passivity, improvement consequences and, 49
Patient appearance
six-week phenomenon and, 17–18
tolerance for, 18–19
Patient Safety Assurance Form, 197, 202
Pedophilia, case illustration, 139–141
Personal appearance, schizophrenia and, 27–29,
33–35
Positive symptoms, schizophrenia
defined, 35–37
impact of, on clinician, 37–41
Positron emission tomography, mental illness and, 184
Post-traumatic process, improvement as, 51–52
Prolixin, 12
Proximate developmental zone, psychotherapy and, 124–126
Psychotherapy, 163–175. *See also* Feelings group
case illustration, 77–85
deinstitutionalization and, 74–77
direction of, 85–86
dissociative personality disorder, 152
effectiveness of, 129–130, 135, 136–138, 142, 143–145
group therapy
background of, 165–166
content and, 171–172
goals of, 168–170
members in, 172
norms and, 170–171
process of, 172–174
topics in, 174
impact of, 86–88
medication group, 166–168
need for, 163–165
proximate developmental zone and, 124–126
violence and, 116–117

Quimby, L. G., 156

Racism
    Clozaril and, 121
    schizophrenia and, 119–121
Recovery, symptoms and,
        190–192
Redner, L., 155
Religion, values and, 182
Risperdal, 8
    described, 188–189
    movement disorders and, 29
Rose, S. M., 155
Ross, C. A., 154, 155
Rudeness, reacting with,
        negative and positive
        symptoms, 41

Sacks, O., 9
Sanity, case histories of reaction
        to, 59–70
Schizophrenia
    Clozaril and, 7–8
    dissociative personality
        disorder and, differential
        diagnosis, 152–157
    etiology of, 108–109,
        182–184
    hallucination and delusion in,
        94–95
    homosexuality and, 115–116
    negative and positive
        symptoms, 35–41
    defined, 35–37
    impact of, on clinician,
        37–41
    neurotransmitters and,
        187–190
    patient history and, 91–94
    personal appearance and,
        27–29, 33–35
    racism and, 119–121

sexuality and, 112–115
spontaneous dyskinesia and,
        21–22
substance abuse and,
        109–110
violence and, 110–112
Schneider, K., 153, 154
Seizures, Clozaril and, 199
Self-concept, improvement
        consequences and, 50–51
Separation, schizophrenia and,
        93
Seroquel, described, 190
Serotonergic receptors, 188
Sertindole, described, 190
Sex role stereotyping
    clinicians and, 112–113
    schizophrenia and, 114
Sexual assault
    case illustration, 135–136,
        141
    psychotherapy and, 136–138
Sexuality
    adolescence, 132
    case illustration, 118, 119
    schizophrenia and, 112–115
    ziprasidone, 190
Sexual molestation
    case illustration, 142
    dissociative personality
        disorder, 154–156
Six-week phenomenon,
        described, 17–18
Smith, T., 156
Social skills, improvement
        consequences and, 49–50
Spaniol, L., 191, 192
Spontaneous dyskinesia,
        described, 19–20
Stable, meaning of, 184–186

Stern, D., 124
Strauss, J. S., 36
Substance abuse
    adolescence, 132
    case illustration, 117–118
    Clozaril and, 200–201
    schizophrenia and, 109–110
Symptoms, recovery and,
    190–192

Tardiff, K., 110, 111
Tardive dyskinesia. *See also*
    Dyskinesia; Movement
    disorders
    Clozaril and, 199–200
    described, 25
Therapeutic relationship
    patient appearance and,
    18–19
    schizophrenia, negative and
    positive symptoms,
    37–41
Thorazine, 12, 19

Tic, described, 26
Titration, of Clozaril, 197–198

Values, religion and, 182
van der Hart, O., 155
van der Kolk, B. A., 51, 155
Violence
    adolescence, 132
    case illustration, 117, 118
    Clozaril and, 122–124,
        133–135
    delusion and, 131
    psychotherapy and, 116–117
    schizophrenia and, 110–112
    sexual assault, 135–136
    sexuality and, 116

Wagner, J., 73, 76
Walker, A., 149

Yassa, R., 19
Yudofsky, S. C., 111

Ziprasidone, 8, 34
    described, 190